Contents

Chapter 1: What is sexual health?

26111

Chapter 2: STIs, HPV and cancer

Chapter 3: Sex education

26111

Introduction

Discussing Sexual Health is Volume 237 in the **ISSUES** series. The aim of the series is to offer current, diverse information about important issues in our world, from a UK perspective.

ABOUT DISCUSSING SEXUAL HEALTH

Sexual health involves more than just being free from sexually transmitted infections (STIs) or not having to face unplanned pregnancy. It means taking responsibility for your body, and your partner's, as well as for your health and the decisions you make about sex. '15 things you should know about sex', 'Contraception myths' and soaring STI rates are just a few of the issues addressed in these pages. This book examines all aspects of sexual health; looking at the possible risks and dangers associated with sex and debating the issue of sex education.

OUR SOURCES

Titles in the **ISSUES** series are designed to function as educational resource books, providing a balanced overview of a specific subject.

The information in our books is comprised of facts, articles and opinions from many different sources, including:

- Newspaper reports and opinion pieces
- Website fact sheets
- Magazine and journal articles
- Statistics and surveys
- Government reports
- Literature from special interest groups

A NOTE ON CRITICAL EVALUATION

Because the information reprinted here is from a number of different sources, readers should bear in mind the origin of the text and whether the source is likely to have a particular bias when presenting information (or when conducting their research). It is hoped that, as you read about the many aspects of the issues explored in this book, you will critically evaluate the information presented.

It is important that you decide whether you are being presented with facts or opinions. Does the writer give a biased or unbiased report? If an opinion is being expressed, do you agree with the writer? Is there potential bias to the 'facts' or statistics behind an article?

ASSIGNMENTS

In the back of this book, you will find a selection of assignments designed to help you engage with the articles you have been reading and to explore your own opinions. Some tasks will take longer than others and there is a mixture of design, writing and research based activities that you can complete alone or in a group.

FURTHER RESEARCH

At the end of each article we have listed its source and a website that you can visit if you would like to conduct your own research. Please remember to critically evaluate any sources that you consult and consider whether the information you are viewing is accurate and unbiased.

D# Health

Independence Educational Publishers

First published by Independence Educational Publishers

The Studio, High Green

Great Shelford

Cambridge CB22 5EG

England

© Independence 2013

Copyright

Photocopy licence

British Library Cataloguing in Publication Data

Discussing sexual health. -- (Issues ; v. 237)
1. Sexually transmitted diseases. 2. Sexually transmitted diseases--Social aspects. 3. Hygiene, Sexual.
I. Series II. Acred, Cara.
616.9'51-dc23
ISBN-13: 9781 86168 635 0

Printed in Great Britain

MWL Print Group Ltd

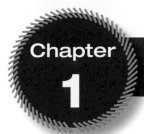

What is sexual health?

Taking care of your sexual health means more than being free from sexually transmissible infections (STIs) or not having to face an unplanned pregnancy. It means taking responsibility for your body, your health, your partner's health and your decisions about sex.

Your body's changing

When you become a teenager, your body changes and develops towards sexual maturity (basically, you go from being a child to an adult). This is called 'puberty'. There are visible changes to your body as well as changes inside. Girls start having periods every month and their breasts grow. For guys, erections become much more frequent and unused sperm is released in semen during a 'wet dream' (usually at night during sleep). Being aware about these changes to your body and knowing they are a normal part of puberty is important.

Being safe with sex

Being safe with sex means caring for both your own health, and the health of your partner. This means being able to talk freely with your partner, both being ready for sex and agreeing on the use of condoms and a suitable type of contraception. Being safe protects you from getting or passing on sexually transmissible infections (STIs) and an unplanned pregnancy. You will enjoy good sexual health if you take care of your genitals (parts of your body that are involved in sex) and avoid any risky behaviour.

Talking about issues related to sex is also important for your mental health and well being. You should feel comfortable talking to your partner and medical professional about anything you are concerned about. Good mental health helps you to enjoy life, enjoy your relationships and enjoy sex.

What is safe sex?

We've all heard the term 'safe sex', but what exactly does it mean?

Being safe with sex means caring for both your own health, and the health of your partner. Being safe protects you from getting or passing on sexually transmissible infections (STIs) and an unplanned pregnancy. Whether you have vaginal, anal or oral sex, it definitely pays to play it safe!

And remember: There's more to sex than sexual intercourse!

There are lots of ways to enjoy physical intimacy with your partner without having oral, vaginal or anal sex. Safe sex also includes lots of other activities like kissing, cuddling, rubbing, massage, stroking, masturbation (touching your own genitals) or touching each other's genitals. Why not explore other ways to be intimate which do not put you at risk of sexually transmissible infections or an unintended pregnancy?

How you can stay safe?

Always use condoms if you have vaginal, oral or anal sex.

Use of condoms is the only method of contraception that protects against both STIs and pregnancy. Even if you're using other methods of contraception (like the pill or a diaphragm), always use condoms as well.

If you are having unprotected sex, talk to your partner about the risks involved. Remember your decision about safe sex is important, as some STIs can be cured but some can't, including HIV (Human Immunodeficiency Virus).

Before having sex, you need to discuss the use of condoms with your partner and come to an agreement about using condoms. Remember, you have the right to say NO if your partner does not agree to use condoms.

Never have sex (even with a condom) if your partner has a visible sore, ulcer or lump on their genitals or anal area. Suggest they see their doctor, family planning clinic or sexual health clinic.

STIs can be passed from one person to another by oral sex. If you put your month in contact with your partner's penis, you need to use a condom to avoid STIs. If you put your mouth in contact with your partner's anus or vulva (outside of vagina) while having sex, you need to use a dental dam (whether you are a guy or girl). This is especially important if you've got a cut or sore around your mouth or lips or bleeding gums.

STIs can also be transmitted if you use sex toys, so you need to be safe. Use condoms and change the condom for each person. Wash the toys carefully after use and wash your hands after removing the condom.

Don't be afraid to talk to your partner about sex.

Contraception

Contraception is a way to prevent pregnancy, and is sometimes called 'birth control'. Some forms of contraception such as condoms can also help reduce the spread of sexually transmissible infections (STIs). Contraception is a very important part of making sure sex is safe and being responsible for your actions.

There are several methods of contraception, including:

⇨ the pill – a tablet taken each day by girls to prevent pregnancy

⇨ condoms – a rubber sleeve worn on the penis

⇨ diaphragms – a rubber device worn inside the vagina

⇨ contraceptive implant (e.g. Implanon) – a device inserted under the skin of girls by a doctor which releases hormones to prevent pregnancy.

'Condoms can also help reduce the spread of sexually transmissible infections'

There is also a form of contraception called the emergency contraception pill, which can help prevent unintended pregnancy. It can be taken by girls within 72 hours after unprotected sex, although preferably within 24 hours. It is available across the counter at chemists or from your local GP, family planning clinic or sexual health clinic.

It's important to talk about contraception with your partner and decide how you will handle any issues before having sex. You both have to be happy with the choice

and make sure you're aware of any risks involved.

Condoms

A condom is a rubber sleeve worn by guys on their penis. Using a condom is very important to help protect you from STIs, including HIV. But remember, some STIs such as genital herpes and genital warts can spread from person to person even when condoms are used.

Tips for using condoms

⇨ Buying correctly. Condoms are available in chemist shops, supermarkets, some petrol stations, and through vending machines. Get the ones that fit you.

⇨ Buying incorrectly. Gimmick shops often sell 'party' condoms. Make sure you only use Australian standard quality approved condoms!

⇨ Storing correctly. Store condoms in a cool, dark place. Only carry them temporarily in your wallet or handbag.

⇨ Storing incorrectly. Keep condoms away from heat (e.g. sunlight) and sharp objects (e.g. ear stud).

⇨ Opening correctly. Tear packet open gently.

⇨ Opening incorrectly. Do not open packet with your teeth, sharp fingernails or scissors.

⇨ Correct lubricants. Always use water-based lubricant.

⇨ Incorrect lubricants. Never use oil-based lubricants.

⇨ Correct condom disposal. Tie the condom in a knot and put it in the bin.

⇨ Incorrect condom disposal. Flushing condoms down the toilet harms the environment.

Other things to remember

⇨ Check the expiry date. Don't use condoms that have expired. Before use, check the condom has not discoloured or become brittle.

⇨ Find the type of condom that suits you and fits well. A condom that's too tight can break and a condom that's too loose can fall off.

⇨ Never use a condom that you have tried to put on inside out as it may have been contaminated. Always use a new condom. Never re-use a condom.

⇨ Some people find certain brands of condoms irritate their skin. Try other brands.

⇨ As fluid may leak out as soon as the penis is hard, put the condom on before the penis goes near your partner's genitals, mouth or anus.

'Don't be afraid to talk to your partner about sex'

What to do if the condom breaks

Stay calm, and withdraw the penis immediately.

Wash the genitals with water (not soap or detergent) and pass urine. Girls shouldn't douche or spray water into their vagina – this can increase the risk of catching a STI.

Once you've removed the condom, be careful not to allow the condom or the penis to touch your partner's genitals, mouth or anus.

Wash your hands after removing the condom.

If there is a risk of pregnancy or exposure to an STI, talk to your local doctor, family planning clinic or sexual health clinic. It's always worth having a check-up.

⇨ The above information is reprinted with kind permission from The State of Queensland. Please visit www.health.qld. gov.au for more information on this and other subjects.

© The State of Queensland (Queensland Health) 2010

15 things you should know about sex

Information from NHS Choices.

1: You can get pregnant the first time that you have sex.

You may have heard that a girl can't get pregnant the first time that she has sex. The truth is, if a boy and a girl have sex and don't use contraception, she can get pregnant, whether it's her first time or she has had sex lots of times.

A boy can get a girl pregnant the first time he has sex. If you're female and have sex, you can get pregnant as soon as you start ovulating (releasing eggs). This happens before you have your first period. Find out more about periods and the menstrual cycle.

Using contraception protects against pregnancy. Using condoms also protects against sexually transmitted infections (STIs). Before you have sex, talk to your partner about contraception, and make sure you've got some contraception. Find out about getting contraception and tips on using condoms.

2: You can get pregnant if a boy withdraws (pulls out) his penis before he comes.

There's a myth that a girl can't get pregnant if a boy withdraws his penis before he ejaculates (comes). The truth is, pulling out the penis won't stop a girl from getting pregnant.

Before a boy ejaculates, there's sperm in the pre-ejaculatory fluid (pre-come), which leaks out when he gets excited. It only takes one sperm to get a girl pregnant. Pre-come can contain sexually transmitted infections (STIs), so withdrawing the penis won't prevent you from getting an infection.

If a boy says he'll take care to withdraw before he ejaculates, don't believe him. Nobody can stop themselves from leaking sperm before they come. Always use a condom to protect yourself against STIs, and also use other contraception to prevent unwanted pregnancy.

3: You can get pregnant if you have sex during your period.

There's a myth that a girl can't get pregnant if she has sex during her period. The truth is, she can get pregnant at any time of the month if she has sex without contraception.

Sperm can survive for several days after sex, so even if you do it during your period, sperm can stay in the body long enough to get you pregnant.

4: You can get pregnant if you have sex standing up, sitting down or in any other position.

You may have heard the myth that a girl can't get pregnant if she has sex standing up, sitting down, or if she jumps up and down afterwards. The truth is, there's no such thing as a 'safe' position if you're having sex without a condom or another form of contraception.

There are also no 'safe' places to have sex, including the bath or shower. Pregnancy can happen whatever position you do it in, and wherever you do it. All that's needed is for a sperm to meet an egg.

5: You can't get pregnant by having oral sex.

You may have heard that you can get pregnant by having oral sex. The truth is, a girl can't get pregnant this way, even if she swallows sperm. But you can catch STIs through oral sex, including gonorrhoea, chlamydia and herpes. It's safer to use a condom on a penis, and a dam (a very thin, soft plastic square that acts as a barrier) over the female genitals if you have oral sex.

6: Drinking alcohol doesn't make you better in bed.

There's a myth that drinking alcohol makes you perform better in bed. The truth is, when you're drunk it's hard to make smart decisions. Alcohol can make you take risks, such as having sex before you're ready, or having sex with someone you don't like. Drinking won't make the experience better. You're more likely to regret having sex if you do it when you're drunk. Find out more about sex and alcohol.

7: You can't use clingfilm, plastic bags, crisp packets or anything else instead of a condom. They won't work

There's a myth that you can use a plastic bag, clingfilm or a crisp packet instead of a condom. The truth is, you can't. Only a condom can protect against STIs.

You can get condoms free from:

⇨   community contraceptive clinics

⇨   sexual health and genitourinary medicine (GUM) clinics

⇨   some young persons services

You can also buy them from pharmacies and shops. Make sure that they have the CE mark on them, as this means that they've been tested to European safety standards. Find sexual health services near you, including contraception clinics.

8: A boy's testicles (balls) will not explode if he doesn't have sex.

You may have heard the myth that if a boy doesn't have sex his balls will explode. The truth is, not having sex doesn't harm boys or girls, and a boy's balls will not explode.

Boys and men produce sperm all the time. If they don't ejaculate the sperm is absorbed into their body. Ejaculation can happen if they masturbate or have a wet dream. They don't have to have sex. Find out about boys' bodies.

9: Condoms can't be washed out and used again.

Don't believe anyone who says that you can wash condoms and use them again. The truth is, you can't use a condom more than once, even if you wash it out. If you've used a condom, throw it away and use a new one if you have sex again.

This is true for male condoms and female condoms. Condoms need to be changed after 30 minutes of sex because friction can weaken the condom, making it more likely to break or fail. Get tips on using condoms.

10: You can get pregnant if you have sex only once.

You may have heard the myth that you have to have sex lots of times to get pregnant. The truth is, you can get pregnant if you have sex once. All it takes is for one sperm to meet an egg. To avoid pregnancy, always use contraception, and use a condom to protect against STIs.

11: You don't always get symptoms if you have an STI.

You may have heard the myth that you'd always know if you had an STI because it would hurt when you pee, or you'd notice a discharge, unusual smell or soreness. This isn't true.

Many people don't notice signs of infection, so you won't always know if you're infected. You can't tell by looking at someone whether they've got an STI. If you're worried that you've caught an STI, visit your GP or local sexual health clinic. Check-ups and tests for STIs are free and confidential, including for under-16s. Find out about sexual health services near you.

12: Women who have sex with women can get STIs.

You may have heard that women who sleep with women can't get or pass on STIs. This isn't true. If a woman has an STI and has sex with another woman, the infection can be passed on through vaginal fluid (including fluid on shared sex toys), blood or close body contact.

Always use condoms on shared sex toys, and use dams to cover the genitals during oral sex. A dam is a very thin, soft plastic square that acts as a barrier to prevent infection (ask about dams at a pharmacist or sexual health clinic). If a woman is also having sex with a man, using contraception and condoms will help to prevent STIs and unintended pregnancy.

13: Not all gay men have anal sex.

You may have heard that all gay men have anal sex. This isn't true. Anal sex, like any sexual activity, is a matter of preference. Some people choose to do it as part of their sex life and some don't, whether they're gay, straight, lesbian or bisexual.

According to the National Survey of Sexual Attitudes and Lifestyles (taken in 2000), 12.3% of men and 11.3% of women had had anal sex in the previous year. Whatever sex you have, use a condom to protect yourself and your partner against STIs. However, having sex isn't the only way to show your feelings for someone.

14: A girl is not ready to have sex just because she's started her periods.

You may have heard that a girl should be having sex once she starts having periods. This isn't true. Starting your periods means that you're growing up, and that you could get pregnant if you were to have sex. It doesn't mean that you're ready to have sex, or that you should be sexually active. People feel ready to have sex at different times. It's a personal decision. Most young people in England wait until they're 16 or older before they start having sex. Find out more about periods and the menstrual cycle.

15: Help is available if you need it.

If you want to talk to someone in confidence, you can call the Sexual Health Helpline on 0800 567 123.

30 September 2011

⇨ The above information is reprinted with kind permission from NHS Choices. Please visit www. nhs.uk for further information.

Sexual health quiz

From www.under-cover.org.uk

1 The contraceptive pill protects against STIs (sexually transmitted infections)?

☐ True
☐ False

2 Lipstick can damage condoms?

☐ True
☐ False

3 If a condom splits during sex a woman has 24 hours to take emergency oral contraception ('the morning after pill')?

☐ True
☐ False

4 Chlamydia can be treated and completely cured?

☐ True
☐ False

5 All STIs have symptoms?

☐ True
☐ False

6 Chlamydia is the most common STI in young people in the UK?

☐ True
☐ False

7 Condoms and femidoms if used correctly and consistently are the only form of contraceptive that will protect you against STIs, HIV/AIDS and unintended pregnancies?

☐ True
☐ False

Answers

1. FALSE – Contraceptive pills do not protect against STIs or HIV/AIDS. They do protect against pregnancy if used correctly.

2. TRUE – Any contact with oil-based products can damage condoms. These include:

– Massage Oils
– Baby Oil
– Sun Tan Creams and Oils
– Cooking Oil
– Ice Cream
– Mayonnaise
– Petroleum Jelly (Vaseline)
– Moisturiser

Water based lubricants are safe to use with condoms.

3. FALSE – The emergency contraceptive pill can be taken within 72 hours. However the sooner it is taken the more effective it is.

4. TRUE – If you test positive for Chlamydia, you will be offered free antibiotics.

5. FALSE – Not all STIs will have symptoms. For example Chlamydia often has no signs or symptoms.

6. TRUE – Chlamydia is the UK's most common curable sexually transmitted infection. It is caused by bacteria and is easily passed on through unprotected anal, oral or vaginal sex or by fingers with an infected person. Chlamydia often has no signs or symptoms.

7. TRUE – Other forms of contraception such as the coil, cap, pill, implant and injection may give some protection against pregnancy but will not protect against sexually transmitted infections.

⇨ The above information is reprinted with kind permission from Bedfordshire PCT. Please visit www.under-cover.org.uk for further information.

© *Bedfordshire PCT*

'Clueless or clued up: your right to be informed about contraception' media report

World Contraception Day 2011.

The 'clueless or clued up: your right to be informed about contraception' media report explores young people's attitudes to sex and contraception, and specifically whether they are able to access accurate and unbiased information about contraception and make informed decisions about their sexual and reproductive health.

The report, written and sponsored by Bayer Healthcare Pharmaceuticals, includes the perspectives of 5,426 young people across 26 countries in Asia Pacific, Europe, Latin America and the USA. 600 young people were also surveyed in Egypt, Kenya and Uganda.

What do the findings tell us?

Young people are still having unprotected sex with new partners for a variety of reasons and knowledge of effective and reliable contraceptive methods is less than optimal. In some countries included in the survey, the situation appears to be getting worse year on year.

In terms of information access, young people appear to be gathering insights about sex and contraception from a wide variety of sources including magazines, the Internet, friends and family as well as from healthcare professionals and school. With the Internet being the overall preferred source of information about sex and contraception, it is also cited as the second most common source of inaccurate information and clearly much of what young people read in social media sites or forums could well be myth or misconception. This is highlighted by the large numbers of young people who believe that ineffective methods of contraception, such as the 'withdrawal method' or having sex during menstruation, will protect them from an unplanned pregnancy.

A considerable number of young people said they have received information on contraception that they have since realised was inaccurate or untrue – in most cases the information was obtained from friends or the Internet but in some cases it was provided by partners or even teachers.

The fact that school does not provide a comfortable environment for questions about sexuality and intimacy was raised as a common barrier preventing young people from being able to obtain accurate and unbiased information on contraception.

In addition to this, the survey results appear to suggest that in some countries there may be a link between poor provision of sex education at school and numbers of unplanned pregnancies, for example in Brazil and Indonesia where there is limited sex education, as many as 67% and 48% of young people have a close friend or family member who has had an unplanned pregnancy. Furthermore, in France and Norway, where 85% and 84% of young people receive sex education, only 25% and 24%, know a close friend or family member who has had an unplanned pregnancy. There is also some correlation between poor provision of sex education and prevalence of misconceptions about effective contraceptive methods – in Turkey and Russia where education provision is low, a large number of young people believe that unreliable methods such as withdrawal or bathing/showering after sex are effective at preventing an unplanned pregnancy.

However, there are exceptions to this, such as in Poland, where 69% of teenagers receive sex education but as many as 56% know someone who has had an unplanned pregnancy. This could suggest that in some countries where there is widespread provision of sex education, the quality of it, in terms of how young people are taught and the topics covered, may vary from school to school and from region to region. Poor services and supplies are also likely to be a factor in the levels of unplanned pregnancies and poor contraception knowledge in some countries, although the survey does not investigate these issues extensively.

No matter where they live, respondents told us that they are too embarrassed to ask for information and that they were unable to access contraception when they needed it because they were too embarrassed to ask a healthcare professional – the very person charged with supplying them with accurate and unbiased information and family planning supplies.

All young people have the right to learn about their sexual and reproductive health and about the importance of asserting one's sexual health rights so they are able to make empowered and informed choices. World Contraception Day 2011, under the theme of 'Live Your Life, Know Your Rights, Learn About Contraception' focuses on the right of young people to access accurate and unbiased information about contraception in order to prevent an unplanned pregnancy or sexually transmitted infection (STI).

Although these survey results report on the incidence of unprotected sex, it is important to note that contraception should always be used to prevent an unplanned pregnancy and/or STI when having sex with a new partner and during a stable relationship.

Did you know...

Young people today

⇨ Nearly half of the world's population (almost three billion people) is under the age of 25[1]

⇨ 44% of young people prioritise personal hygiene, including showering, waxing and applying perfume, above contraception when preparing for a date that may lead to sex[2]

⇨ Studies show that young people do not consider the Internet as the most trustworthy source of information about contraception[3]

1 World Population Foundation website (Last accessed July 2011) http://www.wpf.org/reproductive_rights_article/facts

2 Bayer HealthCare Pharmaceuticals. Data on file. Contraception: Whose responsibility is it anyway? Survey. Fieldwork carried out by GFK Healthcare. May 2010

3 Jones, R., et al, Teens Reflect on Their Sources of Contraceptive Information, Guttmacher Institute 2007

⇨ A young person's mother is the second most trusted source of information about sex and contraception after a doctor. Although, young people feel most comfortable approaching their partner for information[4]

⇨ Embarrassment is a key risk factor in young people's sexual behaviour, this can mean that they resist seeking information and advice about sex and contraception[5]

⇨ School-based sex education delays rather than hastens the onset of sexual activity[6]

⇨ Across the world, inhabitants of 213 countries currently use Facebook[7] – in the countries involved in the WCD 2011 multi-national survey more than 100,000,000 young people (15-19-year-olds) are registered users of the social networking site[8]

4 Bayer HealthCare Pharmaceuticals. Data on file. Talking Sex and Contraception Survey. Fieldwork carried out by TNS Healthcare. July 2009

5 Bell, J. Why embarrassment inhibits the acquisition and use of condoms: A qualitative approach to understanding risky sexual behaviour, J Adolesc. 2009 Apr; 32(2):379-91. Epub 2008 Aug 8

6 Wellings, K., et al, Sexual behaviour in context: a global perspective. The Lancet Sexual and Reproductive Health Series, October 2006

7 Social Bakers online (Last accessed: August 2011) http://www.socialbakers.com/facebook-statistics/

8 Facebook advertising information accessible online (Last accessed: August 2011) http://www.facebook.com/ads/create/

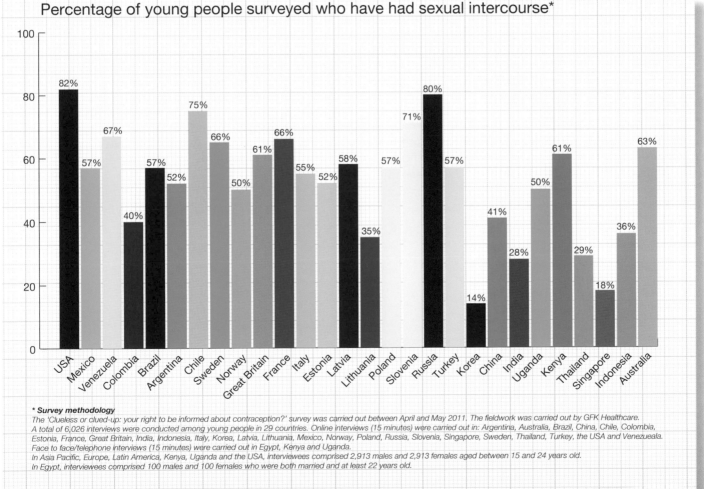

Percentage of young people surveyed who have had sexual intercourse*

USA 82%, Mexico 57%, Venezuela 67%, Colombia 40%, Brazil 57%, Argentina 52%, Chile 75%, Sweden 66%, Norway 50%, Great Britain 61%, France 66%, Italy 55%, Estonia 52%, Latvia 58%, Lithuania 35%, Poland 57%, Slovenia 71%, Russia 80%, Turkey 57%, Korea 14%, China 41%, India 28%, Uganda 50%, Kenya 61%, Thailand 29%, Singapore 18%, Indonesia 36%, Australia 63%

* Survey methodology
The 'Clueless or clued-up: your right to be informed about contraception?' survey was carried out between April and May 2011. The fieldwork was carried out by GFK Healthcare. A total of 6,026 interviews were conducted among young people in 29 countries. Online interviews (15 minutes) were carried out in: Argentina, Australia, Brazil, China, Chile, Colombia, Estonia, France, Great Britain, India, Indonesia, Italy, Korea, Latvia, Lithuania, Mexico, Norway, Poland, Russia, Slovenia, Singapore, Sweden, Thailand, Turkey, the USA and Venezuela. Face to face/telephone interviews (15 minutes) were carried out in Egypt, Kenya and Uganda. In Asia Pacific, Europe, Latin America, Kenya, Uganda and the USA, interviewees comprised 2,913 males and 2,913 females aged between 15 and 24 years old. In Egypt, interviewees comprised 100 males and 100 females who were both married and at least 22 years old.

Source: 'Clueless or clued up: your right to be informed about contraception' media report, 2011, Bayer Health Care Pharmaceuticals © Bayer HealthCare Pharmaceuticals

Incidence of unplanned pregnancies and sexually transmitted infections

⇨ Worldwide, more than 41% of the 208 million pregnancies that occur each year are unintended[9]

⇨ Every year, 14-16 million adolescent females aged 15 to 19 give birth, and pregnancy-related deaths are the leading cause of death for young women this age[10]

⇨ If unmet need for contraception was fully satisfied, each year 53 million more unintended pregnancies could be prevented[11]

⇨ 15% of young adults between the ages of 18 and 26 have had a sexually transmitted disease in the past year[12]

⇨ Ten million women die as a result of pregnancy-related conditions each generation[13]

⇨ One in 20 adolescent girls get a bacterial infection through sexual contact every year and the age at which infections are acquired is becoming younger and younger[14]

⇨ Young adults (15-24 years old) make up only 25% of the sexually active population, but represent almost 50% of all new acquired sexually transmitted diseases[15]

⇨ In 2007, teenagers in the United States were eight times more likely to give birth than teenagers in the Netherlands[16]

⇨ In 2009 there were 38.3 conceptions per thousand women aged 15-17 in England and Wales[17]

Impact of unplanned pregnancies and sexually transmitted infections

⇨ Every £1 invested in contraception saves the UK National Health Service £11 plus additional welfare costs, which is a powerful economic argument for maintaining contraceptive services[18]

⇨ The 1990s witnessed significant gains in access to reproductive health and family planning, but in many less developed countries (LDCs), particularly from Africa, the progress has come to a stand-still since about 2000[19]

⇨ Unplanned pregnancies constitute a global problem associated with substantial costs to health and social services and emotional distress to women, their families and society as a whole[20]

⇨ Having a child early in life may lead to a number of potential disadvantages for both mother and child. Particularly for young teenagers, pregnancy not only carries considerable risks for their health and that of their offspring, but it is also a factor of social, cultural and economic failure[21]

⇨ Children born to teenage mothers are much more likely to experience a range of negative outcomes in later life, such as developmental disabilities, behavioural issues and poor academic performance[22]

⇨ Teen childbearing in the United States costs taxpayers (federal, state and local) at least $9.1 billion annually[23]

⇨ Unintended pregnancy is a key contributor to the rapid population growth that in turn impairs social welfare, hinders economic progress, and exacerbates environmental degradation[24]

⇨ Overall, the cost – just to the National Health Service (NHS) – of teenage pregnancy is estimated to be £69 million annually[25]

⇨ The above information is reprinted with kind permission from Bayer HealthCare Pharmaceuticals. Please visit www.your-life.com for further information.

9   Singh, S., et al. Unintended pregnancy: worldwide levels, trends, and outcomes. Stud Fam Plann (2010)41(4): 241-250

10 Blake, S. et al., Youth Guide for Action on Maternal Health, Women Deliver 2010

11 Global Maternal Mortality Fact Sheet http://www.mothersdayeveryday.org/docs/MDED_FactSheet.pdf

12 Wildsmith, E., et al., Sexually Transmitted Diseases among Young Adults: Prevalence, Perceived Risk, and Risk-Taking Behaviours, Child Trends Research Brief 2010

13 Women deliver website (last accessed May 2011) http://www.womendeliver.org/about/the-issue/

14 WHO 10 facts on sexually transmitted infections, WHO Fact File (Last accessed: August 2011) http://www.who.int/features/factfiles/sexually_transmitted_diseases/facts/en/index2.html

15 Ros et al., Global epidemiology of sexually transmitted diseases. Asian J Androl. 2008 Jan;10(1):110-4.

16 John S. et al., A New Vision for Adolescent Sexual and Reproductive Health, ACT for Youth Center of Excellence

17 Office for National Statistics. Statistical Bulletin. Conceptions in England and Wales 2009.

18 TEENAGE PREGNANCY INDEPENDENT ADVISORY GROUP FINAL REPORT, Teenage pregnancy: Past successes – future challenges

19 Population Dynamics in the Least Developed Countries: Challenges and Opportunities for Development and Poverty Reduction, United Nations population fund, 2011

20 Mavranezouli I et al. Health economics of contraception. Best Practice & Research Clinical Obstetrics and Gynaecology 2009;23:187-198

21 Amy JJ et al. Pregnancy during adolescence: A major social problem. The European Journal of Contraception & Reproductive Health Care. 2007; 12(4): 299-302

22 Hofferth S L et al. Early childbearing and Children's Achievement and Behaviour Over Time. Perspectives on Sexual and Reproductive Health. 2002; 34(1): 41-49

23 NATIONAL CAMPAIGN TO PREVENT TEEN PREGNANCY, By the Numbers: The Public Costs of Teen Childbearing in Texas, http://www.thenationalcampaign.org/costs/pdf/states/texas/fact-sheet.pdf November 2006

24 Speidel, J. et al. Addressing Global Health, Economic, and Environmental Problems Through Family Planning Obstetrics & Gynecology: June 2011 - Volume 117 - Issue 6 - pp 1394-1398

25 Teenage Pregnancy Independent Advisory Group, Annual report 2008 from Teenage Pregnancy Independent Advisory Group http://publicpolicyexchange.co.uk/docs/8J02-PPE_4_Gill_Frances.pdf

Contraception myths

By Kaveh Manavi, for Whittall Street Clinic.

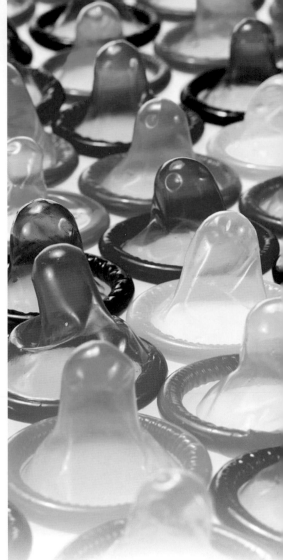

MYTH! 'I don't need contraception because I only have sex during the 'safe' time'

Ovulation (release of egg cell in women) is the result of a delicate balance between four different hormones. Identification of the exact time of ovulation is not easy and requires careful monitoring of several menstrual cycles before using this method. Because of its complexity, this is not a reliable method of contraception. **FACT**

MYTH! 'A woman can't get pregnant if she doesn't have an orgasm'

While the man must ejaculate to release sperm, it is not necessary for the woman to have an orgasm to get pregnant. Ovulation (release of egg) in women can occur without having sex or an orgasm. **FACT**

MYTH! 'I won't get pregnant if we have sex standing up or if I am on top'

The sperm by nature move up through the cervical canal after ejaculation. The woman's position during sex has no effect on the sperm's movement into the womb. Similarly, jumping up and down after sex cannot prevent pregnancy.

MYTH! 'I won't get pregnant if my partner pulls out before he ejaculates'

Pulling out before the man ejaculates is not a reliable method of contraception. Some fluid that contains sperm might be released before the man actually begins to climax. Also, some men might not have the willpower or be able to withdraw in time. **FACT**

MYTH! 'You will not become pregnant if you take a shower or bath right after sex, or if you urinate right after sex'

Washing or urinating after sex will not stop sperm that have already entered through the cervix. **FACT**

MYTH! '"The pill" is effective immediately after you begin taking it'

In most women, one complete menstrual cycle is needed for the hormones in the pill (oral contraceptive) to prevent ovulation. **FACT**

MYTH! 'You can use plastic wrap if you don't have a condom'

Plastic wrap cannot be used as condoms. Condoms are specifically made to provide a good fit and good protection during sex, and they are thoroughly tested for maximum effectiveness. **FACT**

MYTH! 'Toothpaste kills the sperm'

Toothpastes have no effect on the sperm and cannot replace spermicides. **FACT**

MYTH! 'A woman cannot become pregnant if she has sex during her period'

It is true that a woman having her period is not ovulating. The time of ovulation in women may be irregular however. Because sperm can live inside a women's body for five days, a woman who ovulates within seven days of having sex can get pregnant. Having unprotected sex during your period is not a reliable method of contraception. **FACT**

⇨ The above information is reprinted with kind permission from Whittall Street Clinic. Please visit www.whittallstreet.nhs.uk.

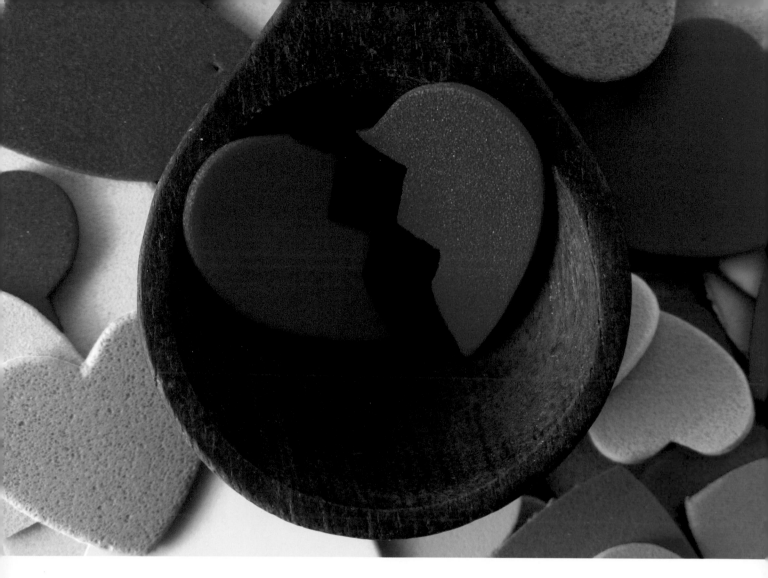

Sexual consent and the law

Information from This is Abuse.

The law

Rape is when a man forces his penis into the vagina, anus or mouth of another person when that person doesn't want him to do so; the law calls this 'without consent'.

The most important bit to remember is that being pressured or forced to have sex when you don't want to is a crime.

Sexual assault is a crime that can be committed by both men and women against men or women. Different types of sexual assault include:

⇨ Objects or parts of the body (e.g. a finger) being put into someone's vagina or anus when that person didn't want it to happen.

⇨ Someone being touched in a sexual way that makes him or her feel uncomfortable or frightened. This could be through their clothes (like bottom pinching).

⇨ Someone being made to sexually stimulate themselves using their hands or fingers (known as masturbation).

⇨ Any other form of physical closeness that happens without consent is known as sexual assault. It can also include; watching other people: having sex, 'sexting' (texting sexual images), and forcing involvement in watching or making pornography.

Consent – what it means

Consent

Consent is someone giving permission or agreeing to something, after they have thought carefully about whether or not they want to do something.

To be able to give your consent you should be sure that it is your decision and not one you have been pressured to make.

The law in Britain says that both people need to give their consent before sex or any physical closeness.

The law also says that to consent to sex a person must be over 16 and have the ability to make informed decisions for themselves.

Being pressured

If you are being forced or pressured into doing sexual things you don't like or aren't sure about, then this is abuse. There are ways someone might try to make you do things without physically forcing you, these can include:

⇨ Being made to feel stupid or bad for saying 'no'.

⇨ Being bullied into having sex.

⇨ Being encouraged to drink lots of alcohol or take drugs to make you more likely to have sex.

⇨ Manipulating your emotions, for example saying 'If you loved me you would...'.

Making sure you have got consent

⇨ Sex with any girl/boy under 16 is unlawful, including oral. It doesn't make any difference if permission (consent) is given or not, if you're under 16 sex is illegal.

⇨ Consent to one sort of sexual activity does not mean you are getting consent to everything. Permission is required for each activity.

⇨ Consent may be withdrawn at any time. If your partner changes their mind, it's their right to do so.

⇨ Even if you have had sex with someone before, you still need permission the next time.

⇨ Giving oral sex to someone without permission is rape.

⇨ If you do not get consent – it's rape.

'Sex with any girl/boy under 16 is unlawful... it doesn't make any difference if permission (consent) is given or not'

More things to look out for to make sure you have consent

When it comes to sex or physical closeness you should feel safe with your partner, be able to trust them and feel that they would respect you whatever your decision.

Good communication between you both will help to ensure you know how your partner feels about sex or physical closeness. It is a good idea to check things out with your partner by asking if they are enjoying what you are doing and asking if they want to continue.

Reading body language is also important. If your partner is relaxed it is likely that they feel comfortable. If they are tense, they may be nervous or frightened and are probably trying to hide how they really feel.

Someone doesn't have to say the word 'NO' to withhold their permission, there are lots of ways they might say they don't want to do something or have sex.

Sometimes people might find it hard to say anything at all if they don't want to have sex, so you should always look out for other signs that they might not be comfortable and might not be giving their consent.

Consequences

What are 'consequences'?

Everything that a person does has an affect on something or someone. This effect is known as a 'consequence'. Consequences can either be positive or negative.

Both positive and negative consequences can have a lasting impact on people's lives.

Sex or physical closeness without consent can have negative consequences for both people involved.

What are the consequences if you have been pressured into sex?

Health

Potential health consequences could include: unwanted pregnancy, sexually transmitted infections for both you and your partner, physical damage, internal injury, mental health problems, depression and self-harm.

Emotional

Potential emotional consequences can include: lower self-esteem and sense of worth, humiliation, fear and hurt.

What are the consequences if you have done the pressuring?

Legal

Having sex without gaining consent could potentially lead to you spending up to eight years in prison.

Sexually assaulting another person could lead to a community order, fine or prison sentence

Both having sex without consent and sexual assault could lead to your details being put on the Sex Offenders' Register.

Health

Potential consequences could include sexually transmitted infections for both you and your partner.

Social

Potential consequences could include being labelled an abuser by people who know you.

What should I do?

Who should I tell if I have been raped or sexually assaulted?

Understand that this was not your fault. There was nothing you could have done to prevent the assault. Nothing you did gave anyone the right to do this. The fault lies entirely with the person who raped or sexually assaulted you.

Firstly, it is important you tell someone as soon as possible and not keep it to yourself. Telling someone what has happened means that you can get the support you need. The person you do talk to should be someone that you trust and feel comfortable with. You may choose to tell: a friend, parent, GP or a school teacher.

You can also speak to the police. Most police forces have specially trained police officers. You can contact the police immediately by dialling 999.

When you talk to the police you will need to give them as much information about the assault as possible, such as what happened, where and when. If you know who assaulted you, tell the police who they are and how you know them. What you tell the police will be recorded in writing or on video and might be used as evidence if your case goes to court.

The police understand how distressing it can be to talk about an assault and will take things slowly. An adult that you trust and feel comfortable with can also support you whilst you are talking to the police.

'It is important you tell someone as soon as possible and not keep it to yourself'

What other help might I be able to get?

You might be given the option to go to a sexual assault referral centre, or SARC. Specialist doctors will ask you about what happened and then examine your body to try and find evidence of what happened to you. Before you go for the examination, try not to shower, wash your clothes, go to the loo (although this may be difficult) or have a drink. Doing so could get rid of evidence, which might be helpful in a police investigation.

The most important thing they do at a SARC is to make sure that you are OK. They will advise you about how to deal with a possible pregnancy, check you for sexually transmitted infections, and sort out treatment if you have caught anything. They can also arrange for you to get support from local services.

The police will talk to you about how a criminal charge can be brought against the person who assaulted you and how they will try and get your case to court.

⇨ The above information is reprinted with kind permission from This is Abuse. Please visit www.thisisabuse.direct.gov.uk for more information on this and other subjects.

© Crown copyright 2012

Myths

MYTH: Only loud or flirtatious girls in tight clothes, or wearing short skirts get raped

FACT: Rape is never the victim's fault. People who are assaulted can be of any age, sex, religion, come from any culture or background and be gay, straight or bisexual.

MYTH: A rapist is likely to be a stranger who rapes someone in a dark alley

FACT: The majority of rapes are committed by people who know and trust each other. They could be friends, partners, family members or know each other from school, college or work.

MYTH: Alcohol and drugs turn people into rapists

FACT: Drugs and alcohol are never the cause of rape or sexual assault. It is the attacker who is committing the crime not the drugs and/or alcohol.

MYTH: When it comes to sex girls say 'no' but they really mean 'yes'

FACT: It's simple – if two people want to have sex with each other it should be something that they both agree and consent to.

MYTH: Rape is only rape if someone gets physically injured

FACT: In some cases people who have been raped have injuries outside or inside their bodies, but not always. Just because someone hasn't got any injuries doesn't mean they weren't raped.

MYTH: It is not rape if the victim does not clearly say 'no'

FACT: Someone doesn't have to say the word NO to withhold permission. There are lots of ways they might say they don't want to have sex. Many people find it hard to say anything, and will show through their body language that they don't want to.

MYTH: Rape is only rape if someone gets physically forced into sex

FACT: This is not true. Rapists often use emotional pressure and manipulative techniques to intimidate and pressure their victims into sex, rather than physical force.

MYTH: If two people have had sex before, it's always OK to have sex again

FACT: This is not true. Just because two people have had sex before it does not mean that consent is not needed the next time they have sex.

MYTH: People often lie about being raped as they regret having sex with someone

FACT: Most people who have been raped or sexually assaulted tell the truth. In fact most people do not tell anyone that they have been raped because they feel too ashamed and scared. Estimates suggest around 8-10% of all rape complaints are false, but there is no evidence to suggest there are more false rape allegations than false allegations of other offences.

Messed up?

Sexual lifestyles of 16-year-olds in Northern Ireland.

By Dirk Schubotz

Introduction

The British National Survey of Sexual Attitudes and Lifestyles (NATSAL) is one of the largest and most comprehensive sexual attitude and lifestyle surveys in the world. The survey takes place approximately every ten years and gives important insights into the sexual health of the British adult population. Very few people now deny that humans are sexual beings from birth and that a healthy sexuality is part of an overall healthy upbringing and lifestyle. With this in mind, studies such as NATSAL provide crucial information not just for health professionals, but for policy makers in general.

Northern Ireland is not included in NATSAL, therefore comprehensive data on if and how the sexual attitudes and lifestyles of people in Northern Ireland differ from the rest of the UK are not available.

However, with funding from the Office of the First Minister and Deputy First Minister of the Northern Ireland Executive (OMDFMNI), sexual health questions were incorporated into the 2011 Young Life and Times (YLT) survey. This article provides a summary of these findings. YLT is an annual study of 16-year-olds in Northern Ireland, undertaken by ARK. Every 16-year-old born in February and March of the survey year who is resident in Northern Ireland and is registered to receive child benefit is invited to take part in the postal YLT survey. In 2011, 1,434 respondents completed the survey, a response rate of 37 per cent.

Sex education

All respondents were asked how easy or difficult they found it to talk about sexual matters to a range of people. As the graph below shows, close friends and boyfriends or girlfriends are the people that

respondents found it easiest to talk to, with nearly two thirds saying this was easy. Around one quarter of respondents found it easy to talk to their mother or sister, if they had one. Only four per cent thought it was easy to talk to their teacher about sexual matters. Despite this unease of talking to teachers about sexual matters, lessons at school were identified as the most helpful source of information about sexual matters (42 per cent of respondents saying this). Thus more than twice as many respnondents rated school lessons as the most helpful source than they did friends (18 per cent), the second most helpful source identified.

Respondents were asked how they would have preferred to get more information about sexual matters. The comments confirmed that school is by far the preferred source of sexuality education, with many respondents saying that they would have liked more lessons in school. As the following quote shows, despite the fact that so few respondents felt at ease talking to their teachers about sexual matters, school lessons were often seen as providing the most reliable information.

'It's good to get sexual information from school because with your friends and the Internet and radio there can be rumours and what they are saying isn't factual, whereas the

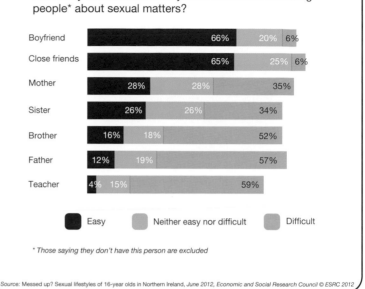

How easy or difficult is it for you to talk to the following people* about sexual matters?

	Easy	Neither easy nor difficult	Difficult
Boyfriend	66%	20%	6%
Close friends	65%	25%	6%
Mother	28%	28%	35%
Sister	26%	26%	34%
Brother	16%	18%	52%
Father	12%	19%	57%
Teacher	4%	15%	59%

* Those saying they don't have this person are excluded

Source: Messed up? Sexual lifestyles of 16-year olds in Northern Ireland, June 2012, Economic and Social Research Council © ESRC 2012

majority of the time school is very factual and it's an important part of life.'

However, some respondents were also critical about the negativity with which sexuality education is taught in school and about the timing of these classes, for example:

'Less stuff on the dangers of sex (pregnancies, STI's) but more on the time when you should have it (in a loving relationship) and explain what happens physically. Don't lecture it and show it in a negative way, it should be positive.'

'More so from school because we only had sex ed in first year when I did not need to know about it because I was not sexually active or interested but now I am [and this] is when I need this advice but there is none on offer.'

Crucially, despite the fact that Relationship and Sexuality Education now forms part of the compulsory post-primary school curriculum, some respondents still reported that they had received none:

'Lessons at school, my year group did not get ANY sexual health education, a disgrace!'

Whether they had had sex or not, respondents were asked whether they would find it easy to access contraception, if they needed any. 62 per cent said they would find this easy. Females and males did not differ significantly in their response to this question

Sexual experience

Around one quarter of respondents (26 per cent) reported that they had had sex. 46 per cent of these were 16 years of age when they did so, 31 per cent were 15 years old whilst the remaining 22 per cent were younger. Proportionately, females were slightly more likely than males to say that they had had sex (28 per cent and 23 per cent respectively). However, among respondents who had had sex, males were much more likely to say that they had done so before they were 16 years of age (61 per cent) than females (49 per cent). 12 per cent of males and two per cent of females who had had sex, said they had sex at least once with a same-sex partner.

Most respondents (81 per cent) who had had sex said they or their partners had used a condom when they first had sex. Nine per cent of all respondents who had had sex said they did not use any means of contraception when they first had sex or they could not remember whether they did.

YLT asked respondents to reflect on the timing of the first time they had sex: 30 per cent said that this had happened on the spur of the moment, whilst 29 per cent said they had planned this together with their partners. Males were much more likely than females to say that it just happened on the spur of the moment (40 per cent and 23 per cent respectively) whilst females were more likely than males to say that they had planned this together with their partner beforehand (31 per cent and 25 per cent respectively). Ten per cent of females but only one per cent of males said that they didn't really want to have sex but felt they should or that they were forced into having sex.

Looking back, 62 per cent of respondents felt that the first time they had sex came at the right time; however, 34 per cent felt it happened too early. Research shows that the older respondents were when they first had sex, the more likely they were to say that the timing was right. Seven out of ten respondents who had sex before they were 14 years of age felt that this was too early. In contrast, nearly three quarters (73 per cent) of those who first had sex at 16 years of age felt that this was the right time.

Respondents were asked for the reasons why they first had sex. Multiple responses were possible in this question. The table below shows that curiosity and the feeling that sex seemed like a natural follow-on to the relationship were the two main reasons why both males and females said they first had sex. The

third most common reason overall given by respondents for having sex was that they were in love, however, females were much more likely to say this (43 per cent) than males (29 per cent). In fact, males were more likely to say that they wanted to lose their virginity (32 per cent) than that they were to say that they were in love (29 per cent). Females and males were equally likely to say that they had sex because everyone else seemed to be doing it (28 per cent and 29 per cent respectively). The graph also shows that more females than males felt not ready to have sex and that only females said they were forced to have sex against their wishes.

Respondents were asked how long the relationship with their first sexual partner continued and how many sexual partners they have had. The lower pie chart on page 17 shows that about one third (31 per cent) of the respondents who had had sex said that they were still in the relationship with this first partner. On the other hand, one in five respondents said that their relationship had not continued at all after they had sex. Females (35 per cent) were much more likely to say that their relationship was still continuing than males (24 per cent). In contrast, males (24 per cent) were more likely than females (17 per cent) to say that their relationship had not continued at all. The earlier respondents said they had sex, the more likely they were to say that the relationship did not continue at all.

As the upper pie chart on page 17 shows, over half of respondents (54 per cent) said they had had one sexual partner only. Only eight per cent of respondents said that they had more than five sexual partners. Females and males did not differ significantly in respect to the number of sexual partners they had.

Just over one in four respondents (26 per cent) who had had sex had used after-sex contraception (or 'emergency contraception'). 16 per cent had used this once, eight per cent two or three times, and two per cent more than three times.

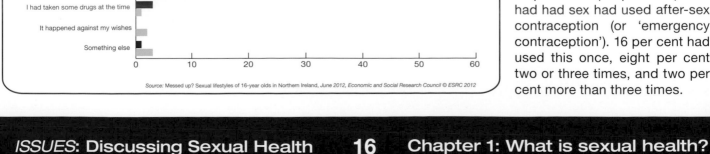

Which of the following things applied to you at the time you first had sex? By gender (%)

- I was curious about what it would be like
- It seemd like a natural follow-on in the relationship
- I was in love
- Most people in my age group seemed to be doing it
- I wanted to lose my virginity
- I was a bit drunk at the time
- I got carried away by my feelings
- I didn't feel ready to have sex, but went along with what the other person wanted
- I had taken some drugs at the time
- It happened against my wishes
- Something else

Males
Females

Source: Messed up? Sexual lifestyles of 16-year olds in Northern Ireland, June 2012, Economic and Social Research Council © ESRC 2012

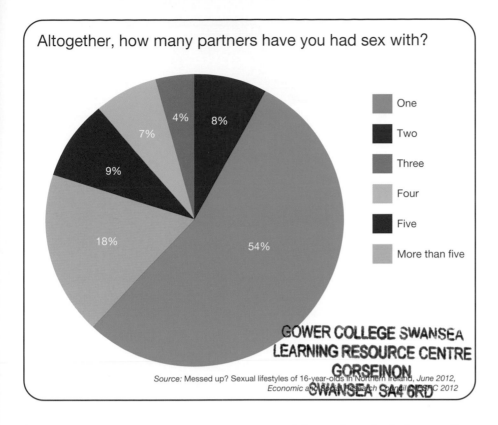

Altogether, how many partners have you had sex with?

- One
- Two
- Three
- Four
- Five
- More than five

8%
4%
7%
9%
18%
54%

Source: Messed up? Sexual lifestyles of 16-year-olds in Northern Ireland, *June 2012, Economic and Social Research Council* © ESRC 2012

Conclusions

The results of the 2011 YLT survey show that nearly three quarters of 16-year-olds had not had sex. Among those who did, almost half said having sex for them was a natural follow-on in the relationship they were in at the time. About one in three had planned their first sexual encounter together with their partner, and three in ten were still in a relationship with their first sexual partner. Looking back, six in ten respondents said that their first sex came at the right time for them. The majority of those who had had sex only had one sexual partner. Eight in ten respondents used a barrier method (condom) when they first had sex which protects them from sexual transmitted infections.

All these findings are myth-busters in the face of those who portray young people as irresponsible, promiscuous, sexed-up beings who don't think much about the consequences of entering a sexual relationship. However, the findings also show that those teaching sexuality education with a 'no sex before marriage' agenda need to acknowledge that many young people don't make this choice. The YLT data clearly show that school-based sex education is young

people's preferred choice as they find this most trustworthy. However, in order not to fail young people, the YLT findings suggest that a more open and positive approach is required for this.

Apart from the standard of sex education, there are some other reasons for concern. The findings clearly show that the later respondents have sex the less

they are likely to regret this and the more they are likely to be in a stable relationship with their partner. One third of males also said they had sex because they wanted to lose their virginity, which would be an indication that especially young males may still experience pressure from their peer group to have sex. As one respondent commented:

'I know a number of 12-14-year olds who are already considering to have sex simply because their friends have said they had.'

So, is the sexual health of 16-year-olds in Northern Ireland just 'messed up' as one 16-year-old felt? Whilst there is little reason to be as negative as some of the respondents were themselves, there is no room for complacency and still much more work to be done so that young people feel they can openly discuss sexual matters with adults.

June 2012

⇨ The above information is reprinted with kind permission from ARK. Please visit www.ark.ac.uk for further information.

© 2012 ARK

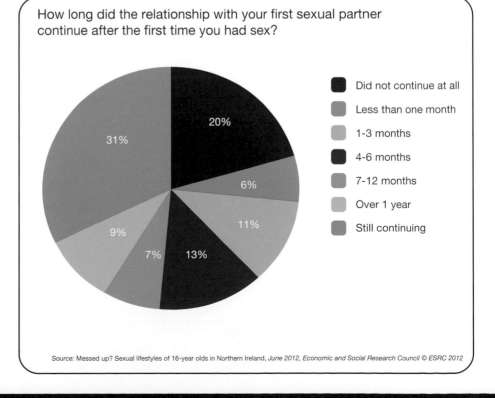

How long did the relationship with your first sexual partner continue after the first time you had sex?

- Did not continue at all
- Less than one month
- 1-3 months
- 4-6 months
- 7-12 months
- Over 1 year
- Still continuing

20%
6%
11%
13%
7%
9%
31%

Source: Messed up? Sexual lifestyles of 16-year olds in Northern Ireland, *June 2012, Economic and Social Research Council* © ESRC 2012

All about STIs

Information from Brook.

What is an STI?

An STI, or sexually transmitted infection, is basically any kind of bacterial or viral infection that can be spread through sexual contact.

This doesn't just mean unprotected sex. Some STIs can be passed on through oral sex (kissing, licking or sucking someone's genitals), and some can be passed through sexual touching and skin-to-skin contact.

'The best way to avoid STIs is to use a condom every time you have sex'

There are lots of STIs out there and you will probably already have heard of some like chlamydia, gonorrhoea, genital warts, genital herpes, HIV...

Many are on the increase, and all of them can affect anyone. Some don't show up straight after you get infected.

Some can show signs a few days after unprotected sex. Others can go unnoticed for a long period of time. Some don't ever show any symptoms at all.

The good thing about infections is that they're often easy to sort out. But leave them untreated and they may cause serious damage to your long-term health.

How to avoid STIs

The best way to avoid STIs is to use a condom every time you have sex.

STIs are usually passed on by sex with an infected person, although some infections can be passed on in other ways as well. STIs can be caught during oral (licking, kissing or sucking someone's genitals), vaginal or anal sex and some can also be passed through sexual touching and skin-to-skin contact.

Even if you're using other kinds of contraception to prevent pregnancy, like the pill, you should still use a condom as well. Using a condom every time you have sex is the only way to protect yourself from STIs as well as pregnancy. If you have any questions about using condoms, contact Ask Brook on 0808 802 1234. Your call will be confidential. That means we won't tell anyone about it.

'Many STIs have similar symptoms. Some don't have any at all'

Condoms and dental dams

Some STIs, such as genital warts and herpes, can be passed on through skin-to-skin contact, so although condoms and dental dams can't protect against all STIs,

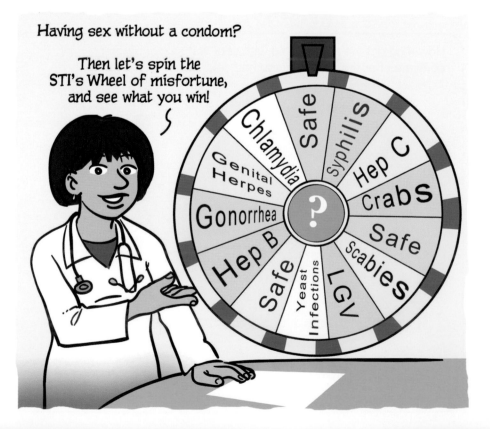

they are still the most effective way to reduce the risk of picking up, or passing on an infection – including HIV.

'Keep an eye open for tell-tale signs and be ready to ask for advice and help if you need to'

Use a condom for vaginal sex, anal sex or oral sex. Male or female condom, it doesn't matter, they both work. A condom acts as a barrier and stops body fluids from mixing during vaginal, oral or anal sex.

Dental dams are small squares of latex which work well as a barrier during sex involving contact between the mouth and the vagina, or mouth and the anus.

You can get FREE condoms from all kinds of places:

⇨ Brook Centres

⇨ Other young people's clinics

⇨ Family planning centres or CASH (Contraception and Sexual Health) clinics

⇨ GUM clinics.

Or buy your condoms from:

⇨ Chemists

⇨ Petrol stations

⇨ Machines in public toilets, bars and clubs.

'Even if you're using other kinds of contraception to prevent pregnancy, like the pill, you should still use a condom'

Signs and symptoms of STIs

Many STIs have similar symptoms. Some don't have any at all. So dont even think about diagnosing or treating yourself without talking to someone who is trained.

Keep an eye open for tell-tale signs and be ready to ask for advice and

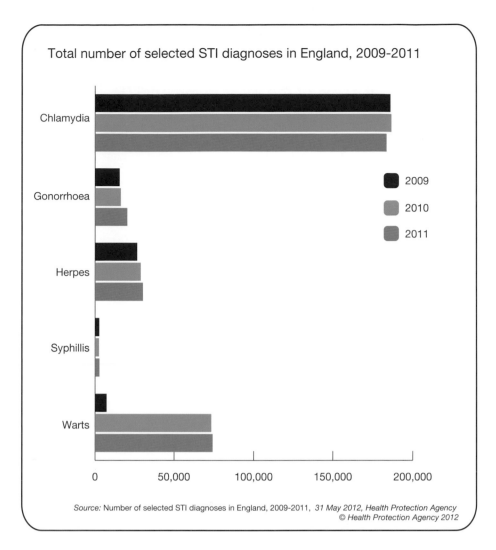

Total number of selected STI diagnoses in England, 2009-2011

Source: Number of selected STI diagnoses in England, 2009-2011, *31 May 2012, Health Protection Agency*
© Health Protection Agency 2012

help if you need to. If you're at all worried, it might even be a good idea to have a check-up anyway just to be sure you're in the clear. If you want to talk to someone, you can always contact Ask Brook on 0808 802 1234. Your call will be confidential. That means we won't tell anyone about it.

You can find out about the particular symptoms of individual STIs in the Types of STIs section on www.brook.org.uk but to help you, here are some common symptoms to look out for...

Men

⇨ Discharge from the penis

⇨ Sore, tender or inflamed penis head

⇨ Testicle ache or pain

Women

⇨ Unusual vaginal discharge – a change in texture or colour

⇨ Bleeding in between periods

⇨ Sore, tender or inflamed vulva

'You can get FREE condoms from all kinds of places'

Men or women

⇨ Stinging sensation when you urinate

⇨ Itching, blisters or sores in the genital region. Also the mouth.

⇨ Pain during sex

⇨ Anal discharge or itching

⇨ Feverish, flu-like symptoms with any of the above

⇨ The above information is reprinted with kind permission from Brook. Please visit www.brook.org.uk

© Brook

Types of STIs

Details about some of the most common STIs.

Chlamydia

The most common STI in the UK is chlamydia. The infection is caused by bacteria that can infect your cervix (the neck of your womb), urethra (the tube that carries urine from your bladder and out through your penis or vulva), rectum (back passage), throat or eyes.

'If you get infected with HPV, you may get warts on your genitals and anal area.'

About seven in ten infected women and half of infected men won't have any obvious signs or symptoms of chlamydia. If you do have signs or symptoms, these usually show up one to three weeks after being infected or may show many months later when the infection has spread to other parts of your body. Possible symptoms in women can include:

⇨ bleeding between periods or heavier periods

⇨ pain and/or bleeding during or after sex

⇨ lower abdominal pain

⇨ unusual vaginal discharge – such as a change in colour, texture or smell

⇨ pain when passing urine.

Symptoms in men can include:

⇨ a white, cloudy or watery discharge from the tip of the penis

⇨ pain when passing urine

⇨ pain in the testicles.

You may have symptoms in other areas of your body and some of these symptoms can be similar to other diseases, such as arthritis (joint pain). If you have an infection in your rectum, you may notice an unusual discharge from your anus and you may have pain there. You may get conjunctivitis, an inflammation of the transparent surface layer that covers the white of the eye (the conjunctiva).

Chlamydia can be treated with antibiotics. This may either be a single dose of an antibiotic or a course of antibiotics. If you have the signs and symptoms of chlamydia, you may be given treatment before your test results are back.

Genital warts

Genital warts, the second most common STI in the UK, are caused by infection with human papilloma virus (HPV). If you get infected with HPV, you may get warts on your genitals and anal area. Warts can vary in appearance. They can appear as small, smooth, round bumps or larger growths that are grouped together or small cauliflower-shaped bumps. Genital warts can also grow inside your urethra, vagina and anus. You can have HPV without having any symptoms, and you can pass on the virus even when you don't show any signs of having genital warts. Using condoms reduces the chances of you passing on the virus but, as the infected areas of skin might not be covered by a condom, this may not fully protect you or your partner against genital warts.

Although the warts may disappear on their own, you can be treated with a chemical solution or liquid nitrogen (cryotherapy) to remove them faster. Surgery or laser treatment are also options. You may need to have repeat treatment to get rid of the warts.

Genital herpes

Genital herpes is caused by the herpes simplex virus. Many people infected by this virus won't have any symptoms. If you do have symptoms, you may first notice stinging, tingling or itching in the genital or anal area followed by the development of fluid-filled blisters or sores on your genitals, anal area or tops of your thighs. You may also feel generally unwell, tired or have a fever.

The blisters will heal within about three weeks, but after the first 'primary' episode of genital herpes, you may have further outbreaks in the coming months. These outbreaks tend not to last as long or be as severe.

Another type of the virus causes oral herpes (cold sores). These can be passed to the genitals during oral sex. Genital herpes can also be passed to the mouth by oral sex.

'Gonorrhoea is caused by bacteria that can infect your urethra, cervix, rectum, mouth and throat'

There is no treatment that can completely remove the virus from your body, but you can be prescribed antiviral medicine by your GP that will help to clear up the blisters more quickly. You may be able to manage your symptoms by having salt baths and taking painkillers. You can have the virus but not show any symptoms and still pass the virus on to your partner. Using condoms can help to lower the chances of passing the virus on, but can't completely prevent this happening.

Gonorrhoea

Gonorrhoea is caused by bacteria that can infect your urethra, cervix, rectum, mouth and throat. You may have symptoms that appear up to 14 days after you become infected. However, one in ten men and half of all women who are infected have no symptoms.

In women, symptoms may include:

⇨ unusual vaginal discharge, which may be yellow or green

⇨ pain when passing urine

⇨ lower abdominal pain or tenderness (this is rare)

⇨ rarely, bleeding between periods or heavier periods.

In men, symptoms may include:

⇨ unusual discharge from the tip of the penis, which may be white, yellow or green

⇨ pain when passing urine

⇨ rarely, pain or tenderness in the testicles

⇨ inflammation of the foreskin (this is less common).

You may sometimes have other symptoms depending on where the infection is. If it's in your rectum, usually there aren't any symptoms but you may have anal pain, discomfort or discharge. If you have the infection in your throat, you usually won't have any symptoms.

It's important to be treated for gonorrhoea as the infection can cause serious long-term health problems including infertility. Gonorrhoea can be treated with antibiotics.

Hepatitis B

Hepatitis B virus causes hepatitis, which is an inflammation of your liver. If you have any symptoms, and not everyone does, these start about one to six months after you become infected. You may feel generally unwell with a sore throat, tiredness, joint pains and a loss of appetite. You may also feel sick or vomit. Your symptoms may be more severe and cause abdominal pain and yellowing of your skin and eyes (jaundice). Your skin may itch and your urine may become darker.

Most people will recover from hepatitis B without treatment, but if you don't clear the infection after six months, you will become a chronic carrier of the disease. Being a chronic carrier means you may have no symptoms and be unaware that you're infected, but you can still pass the infection on to other people. A chronic illness is one that lasts a long time, sometimes for the rest of the affected person's life. When describing an illness, the term 'chronic' refers to how long a person has it, not to how serious a condition is. Being a chronic carrier means you will be at a greater risk of developing cirrhosis of the liver and liver cancer.

You may be treated for hepatitis B with medicines including antivirals or ones that help your immune system fight the disease. A vaccine is also available to prevent hepatitis B. If you haven't been vaccinated against hepatitis B and have been exposed to the virus through sexual contact with someone who has the virus, you can be given an injection (hepatitis B immunoglobulin) and an accelerated course of the vaccine. You would be given this treatment at a sexual health clinic. It works best if you are given this within 48 hours of exposure.

HIV

Human immunodeficiency virus (HIV) attacks your immune system. Many people infected with HIV have no signs and symptoms at all. About half of people who become infected with HIV will have flu-like symptoms within a few weeks of becoming infected.

There is currently no treatment that can get rid of HIV from your body. However, at specialist centres, you can be given a combination of antiretroviral medicines to reduce the level of HIV in your blood. These treatments are very effective and work best if started sooner rather than later. It's important to be treated for HIV to reduce your risk of having serious health complications later on. Even if you're taking antiretroviral medicines for HIV, you can still pass on the infection through unprotected sex. If you have had unprotected sex with someone who has HIV or is at high risk of having HIV, you will be offered the option of taking a month's course of antiretroviral medicines (this is called post-exposure prophylaxis) to lower the chances of developing the infection. These work best if started as soon as possible after exposure. Accident and emergency departments and sexual health clinics are the best places to get post-exposure prophylaxis.

Pubic lice

Pubic lice (also known as crabs) are tiny insects that live in coarse body hair such as pubic hair but also chest and leg hair, beards, eyelashes and eyebrows. They don't live in hair on the head and are not the same as head lice.

You may notice the lice in your body hair, but they are very tiny and hard to see. Other signs include finding the brown eggs (nits) stuck to your body hair, or seeing black powdery spots in your underwear from the lice droppings. Pubic lice may make you itch.

You can treat a pubic lice infection with lotions or shampoos that you may need to use over your whole body or leave on for up to 12 hours.

Syphilis

Syphilis is caused by bacteria. The disease has three stages: primary, secondary and tertiary. The primary stage begins about two to three weeks after you are infected when one or more sores may appear. Commonly these develop on your penis, anus, in your vagina or rectum, in your mouth or on your lips.

The secondary stage begins a few weeks after the sores have healed. You may have symptoms including feeling generally unwell with flu-like symptoms and a rash. If you aren't treated for syphilis, you can develop the tertiary stage of the disease. This can cause serious health problems including problems with the nervous system and heart.

Syphilis can be treated with antibiotics.

November 2011

⇨ Content provided by Bupa. For more information visit www.bupa.co.uk/health.

© Bupa 2011

Chlamydia

Information from Test Me.

Chlamydia is the most common sexually transmitted infection amongst young people.

One in ten who have a chlamydia test find they are infected!

Most people wouldn't even know if they had it because most of the time chlamydia shows no symptoms. Yet left untreated chlamydia can lead to serious health problems and is the most common cause of infertility.

Signs and symptoms of chlamydia

75% of women and 50% of men show no symptoms.

If there are any symptoms, they could include:

Symptoms in women

⇨ Increased vaginal discharge.

⇨ Pain during sex.

⇨ Bleeding after sex.

Symptoms in men

⇨ Discharge from the penis.

⇨ Pain/burning sensation when you go for a pee.

⇨ Painful swelling of the testicles if left untreated.

How do you get chlamydia?

⇨ Penetrative sex (where the penis enters the vagina or anus).

⇨ Oral sex (from mouth to the genitals).

⇨ Mother to baby during birth.

⇨ Occasionally by touching the eyes after touching the genitals.

Risks of chlamydia

If you have chlamydia and it's not treated, the infection can spread in your body and can cause health problems. Not everyone who has chlamydia will develop these complications, but the risk increases the more times you get infected.

In men and women

If left untreated chlamydia can cause Reiter's syndrome, a form of arthritis which causes swelling of the joints, inflammation of the urethra (the tube which carries your wee from your bladder) and the eyes.

In women

If left untreated, chlamydia can lie dormant for several months before travelling through the cervix to infect the fallopian tubes leading to Pelvic Inflammatory Disease (PID). This can cause symptoms such as low abdominal pain, fever and painful sex. Many women have a less serious inflammation that produces few, if any symptoms. If untreated, PID can lead to blockage of the fallopian tubes which can result in infertility or may cause an ectopic pregnancy which can be very serious and even life-threatening.

Chlamydia is now the commonest cause of PID, which is thought to affect more than 165,000 women a year. It is estimated that 25% of all cases of infertility are due to chlamydia infection.

Approximately 10% of all women who contract chlamydia will become infertile as a result of PID. This equates to around 30,000 women a year becoming infertile.

In men

Chlamydia can cause painful inflammation in one or both testicles. It's thought that chlamydia may also lead to reduced fertility or infertility in men; however, less is known about whether this happens.

A study in 2007 revealed that men carrying the infection produced sperm with 80% more physical abnormalities and 10% less mobility. Following treatment it was found that the DNA damage in the men's sperm had typically fallen by over 35%.

About the test

The information below relates to the freetest.me test kit that we use. If you're referred to a local NHS website to request your kit then it may vary slightly.

It's quick and simple to complete your chlamydia test and return it to our laboratory.

What will arrive

Once you've completed the Chlamydia test request, your test will arrive in the mail in discreet packaging.

The kits are small, around the size of a couple of DVD cases and contain all the bits you need to return your sample to our laboratory, including free return postage.

How to take your sample

Your test will require either a urine sample, or a vaginal swab.

Once you've taken your sample, ensure you have completed the included form (but keep the top part – you may need it to collect your results).

Place your sample and the form back in the box, remove the adhesive strip and seal the box shut. Post the box as soon as you can – a normal post box is fine.

Result notification

You will receive your results via the method you chose when requesting the chlamydia test. You may also track your specimen and collect results any time via our tracking system.

2010

⇨ The above information is from Test Me. Please visit www. freetest.me.uk for further information.

© *test.me 2010*

New survey reveals young people are unaware of STI risks

A new survey of 16-to-25 year-olds has revealed a worrying lack of concern about the dangers of STIs, with almost half (47%) of respondents agreeing that it's OK to have sex without a condom, providing the girl is on the pill.

The survey, which was part of a wider project looking into young people's attitudes towards sex and alcohol for TheSite.org, also revealed that one in three (29%) of respondents caught an STI after a night of drinking and 62% of respondents who had unprotected sex didn't go for an STI test afterwards.

Dr Ranj Singh, an expert in young people's health said: 'It's alarming to see such relaxed attitudes towards condom use amongst young people, but more importantly indicates that there's a significant lack of awareness of the risks associated with contracting STIs.

'Figures for the number of young people infected with STIs are at record highs and this problem is not going away, so it's absolutely essential that we look at ways of ensuring young people are clear about the facts.'

Other results from the survey showed that over a third (36%) of respondents had obtained emergency contraception after a night of drinking, 58% had kissed or had sex with someone they wouldn't normally fancy and 48% had a one night stand they regretted.

Emma Thomas, CEO at charity YouthNet, which runs TheSite.org said: 'It's understandable that many young people will experiment with sex and alcohol as part of their transition to adulthood, yet it's vital that they recognise the risks.

'The results of the survey show that there is still some way to go in helping them understand the myriad of dangers of unprotected sex.

'By continuing to evolve the advice and support available through TheSite.org as well as meeting the needs of young people through new technology and platforms, we can ensure more young people have the right information wherever and whenever they need it, helping them with the confidence to make informed decisions.'

TheSite.org, run by charity YouthNet, offers straight-talking information, advice and guidance on anything and everything a young person might need to know – from drink and drugs, to housing, tax, relationships and emotional well-being. It also features an expert question and answer service and a thriving moderated community offering instant peer support.

About the research

Between the 5 December 2011 and 9 February 2012, YouthNet conducted an online survey completed by 719 16-to 25-year-old residents of the UK.

The survey explored young people's attitudes and behaviours relating to alcohol and sex, with a specific focus on their help-seeking behaviour when it came to issues emerging from a night out drinking.

Because of self-selection issues, the sample is fully NOT representative of young people in the UK.

The full report can be viewed at www.youthnet. org/2012/04/young-people-unaware-of-sti-risks/

⇨ Total respondents: 719 young people aged 16-25 from the UK

⇨ Base – Only respondents who have had sex and got drunk enough to lose control at least once in their life: 560

⇨ Base – Only respondents who have had sex and got drunk enough to lose control at least once in their life: 560

⇨ Base – Only respondents who had unprotected sex: 169

⇨ Base – Only respondents who have had sex and got drunk enough to lose control at least once in their life: 560

⇨ Base – Only respondents who have had sex and got drunk enough to lose control at least once in their life: 560

⇨ Base – Only respondents who have had sex and got drunk enough to lose control at least once in their life: 560

24 April 2012

⇨ The above information is reprinted with kind permission from YouthNet. Based on research by YouthNet, the charity behind www.thesite. org, which offers support and information on sex, relationships, drugs, work, study and health to 16-25 year olds in the UK. Please visit www.youthnet. org for further information.

Sexually transmitted infection rates soar among young

Gonorrhoea cases causing major concern as health agency warns under-25s failing to use condoms with new partners.

By Sarah Boseley

Sexually transmitted infections are soaring among young people failing to use condoms with new partners, the Heath Protection Agency warns. There is particular concern about the numbers of very young people contracting gonorrhoea. Over half of all new infections – 57% – are in the under-25s, said the HPA in its annual report for England. Gonorrhoea cases among girls increased sharply from the age of 15 to peak at the age of 18, said Dr Gwenda Hughes, head of STI surveillance. 'We have got high rates of infection in this population. In the older group it is much lower – particularly in women,' she said.

There is also major concern about men who have sex with men – who may be gay or bisexual. The largest upsurge in new diagnoses in 2011 were among this group. Gonorrhoea cases increased by 61%, chlamydia by 48% and syphilis by 28%. Sexual health charities suggested the Government's policy of cutting funding for sexual health awareness campaigns could be a factor while the Department of Health said more people were coming forward to be tested.

'The data in young, heterosexual people and MSM is very concerning,' said Hughes. 'Too many people are practising unsafe sex. They are getting STIs and putting themselves at risk of longer-term problems, such as [in women] ectopic pregnancies and tubal infertility. We think it is crucial that work to reduce STIs continues with a focus on at-risk groups.'

In 2011, the number of newly diagnosed STIs rose by 2%, totalling nearly 427,000 new cases and reversing the small decline seen in previous years.

While the Government believes that more and better testing is a factor in the overall rise, HPA experts said they were worried to see a downturn in the number of people coming for a chlamydia test. Dr Angie Bone, director of the HPA's national chlamydia screening programme, said the numbers of diagnoses had dropped from 154,000 in 2010 to 148,000 last year, which did not mean less chlamydia in the community but less testing. 'This is something we are very keen to reverse,' she said. Chlamydia is a very common infection that often has no symptoms, but left untreated it can cause infertility.

Sexually active young people and MSM are recommended to have a chlamydia test every year and whenever they change partners. MSM should also have an HIV test with the same frequency. 'The more partners you have, the greater the risk of getting an STI,' said Hughes. 'People should consider reducing the number of partners they have and reduce overlap in their sexual partnerships.'

Gonorrhoea is becoming a bigger worry because the drugs used to treat it are losing their effect. 'This is a global problem, not just a UK problem,' said Hughes. 'This bug has successfully managed to develop resistance to every treatment that has been used for it for a decade. We are running out of options for managing this infection. We are concerned in the future it will become very difficult to treat.'

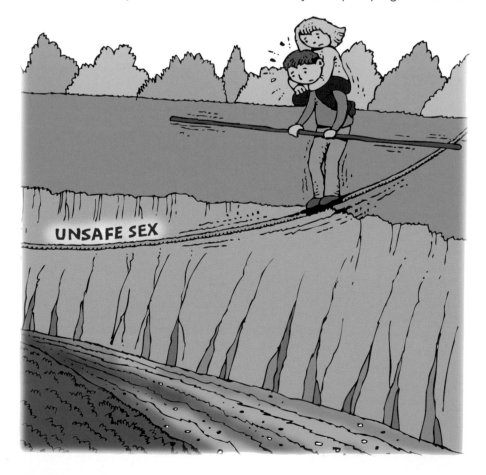

UNSAFE SEX

There were 20,065 cases of gonorrhoea last year, which is a 25% rise on the 16,835 in the previous year and the biggest rise in any STI. Syphilis cases were up 10% from 2,650 to 2,915. Genital herpes and warts were also up by 5% and 1%, respectively. Chlamydia was down 2% from 189,314 to 186,196 cases.

There is concern that advertising campaigns and efforts to increase people's awareness of the risks of STIs have decreased. The last chlamydia awareness campaign, called 'Sex worth talking about', was in 2010. When the Coalition Government came to power, it temporarily froze all spending on social marketing, although funding for campaigns such as the anti-obesity drive Change4Life has resumed. The onus under the health reforms will now be on local authorities, who will be expected to champion the public health initiatives needed in their own area.

Sexual health charities FPA and Brook said in a joint statement that the rise in STIs is a worrying trend. 'It demonstrates exactly why safer sex messages and campaigns that young people and gay men will listen to and take action on, are absolutely necessary. Testing and treatment services are vital, but alone they are not enough to change people's behaviour.

'The impact of the Government's disinvestment in campaigning around safer sex and sexual health reflects in today's statistics. Yet again we see more data illustrating why there is an urgent need for statutory sex and relationships education in schools alongside sustained investment in sexual health services.'

A Department of Health spokesperson said: 'The fact that more people are coming forward to be tested and the improvements there have been in the way tests are done is to be welcomed.

But it's also clear that not enough people are taking care of their sexual health.

'Sexually transmitted infections can lead to infertility and other serious health problems. The message is clear: whatever your age, you should always use a condom.

'We are changing the way we deal with public health issues by giving local councils ring-fenced budgets so they can raise awareness of and improve sexual health in their communities.'

31 May 2012

⇨ The above article originally appeared in *The Guardian* and is reprinted with permission. Please visit www.guardian.co.uk for further information.

Condoms: too embarrassed to buy them?

Extracts from YouGov Labs discussions.

Male participants who were not embarrassed to buy condoms

A recurring opinion emerged; buying condoms is a 'mark of pride', not something to be uncomfortable about:

'Why should the cashier care? I see it almost as a mark of pride' *Inverness*

'We all know what they are for, so why be embarrassed? We should be proud that we're having safe sex' *Robert Portland Dorset*

Male participants who were embarrassed to buy condoms

A small number of male participants said they were embarrassed to buy condoms. One reason was because they have experienced – or felt that people judge them:

'Because people sometimes give you dirty looks' *Anon*

To some participants buying condoms seemed like a public statement that one is planning to have sex, which is usually hidden:

'You are effectively saying to everyone who can see you, I plan on having sex. We usually hide this statement, or wrap it up with lots of jokes and euphemisms' *Anon*

Female participants who were not embarrassed to buy condoms

More female participants said they were not embarrassed to buy condoms, than embarrassed. Many believed that buying condoms is normal and that it doesn't actually imply that one is sleeping around:

'It's a normal thing, plus it's possible to be in a relationship and buy condoms regularly so it doesn't mean you're sleeping around. Not that the shop assistants care anyway' *Anon*

Females also outlined the health factor and said that buying condoms is the responsible thing to do. Unlike men participants, they seemed to mention the function of protecting from unplanned pregnancy more:

'I prefer buying condoms to getting pregnant and/or getting a disease' *Anon*

'It would be embarrassing if you caught a disease from not wearing one, so better safe than sorry!' *Una, Cardiff*

'I am not embarrassed as I think it should be looked upon as taking responsibility of unwanted child or risk of infection' *Sue*

Female participants who said they were embarrassed to buy condoms

Only a small number of female Labs participants said they were embarrassed to buy condoms. The main reason was feeling judged:

'As a female from an Asian background, I feel I will be judged by the sales person, the cashier and also the people around me' *Anon*

9 November 2012

⇨ Information from YouGov. www.yougov.co.uk.

HPV vaccines

Can you tell me about the vaccine to prevent HPV (human papilloma virus)?

What the human papilloma virus (HPV) is

There are over 100 different types of human papilloma virus (HPV). It is sometimes called the wart virus or genital wart virus because some types of HPV cause genital warts. A number of HPV types are passed on from one person to another through sexual contact. Many women will be infected with the HPV virus at some point during their lifetime. Often the virus causes no harm and goes away without treatment.

HPV and cancer

Some types of HPV can increase the risk of developing cervical cancer. Cervical cancer is cancer of the neck of the womb. Almost 3,400 women are diagnosed with this type of cancer every year in the UK. Most women infected with

HPV don't go on to develop cervical cancer. But for some, infection with HPV can go on to cause

⇨ Genital warts

⇨ Changes in the cervix, which may develop into cervical cancer

⇨ Changes in the vaginal tissues, which may develop into vaginal cancer.

Of the different types of HPV, types 16 and 18 cause about seven out of ten (70%) cancers of the cervix. Most of the remaining 30% of cervical cancers are associated with other high-risk HPV types. HPV types 6 and 11 cause genital warts but are rarely linked to cancer. HPV is also a risk factor for other types of cancer including vulval cancer, anal cancer, cancer of the penis and mouth and oropharyngeal cancers.

Research into vaccines to prevent HPV

Several research trials have tested vaccines as a way of preventing infection with HPV. There are two cervical cancer vaccines, Gardasil and Cervarix. A trial testing Gardasil called FUTURE II reported its results in October 2005. This phase three trial involved over 12,000 women aged between 16 and 26. These women did not have HPV before the start of the trial. The women were divided into two groups. Half the women were given Gardasil and the other half had a dummy vaccine (placebo). Both groups of women had three injections of either the vaccine or placebo over six months.

Over the following two years the women had regular checks to see if they had got HPV, or had any pre-cancerous changes to the cells of the cervix, which could develop into a cancer. The group who had the vaccine showed no pre-cancerous changes. Of the 5,258 women who had the placebo, 21 had pre-cancerous changes, which is 0.4%. The researchers found that Gardasil protected against HPV types 6 and 11 (which cause about 90% of genital warts), as well as 16 and 18. Gardasil was licensed in the UK in September 2006 for girls and women aged between nine and 26.

Two phase three trials have tested the vaccine Cervarix. The first was for women under 26. It involved over 18,000 women from all over the world, including the UK. This study was called PATRICIA (PApilloma TRIal to prevent Cervical cancer In young Adults). The second was for women of 26 and over. The trials found that Cervarix was useful in preventing HPV infection. Cervarix was licensed in the UK in 2007 for the prevention of pre-cancerous changes in the cervix in girls and women between the age of ten and 25.

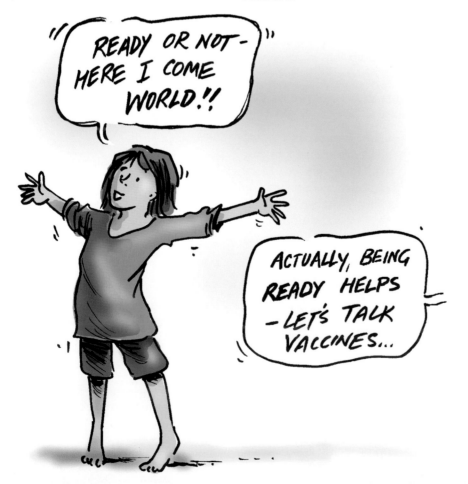

There is not enough evidence at the moment that the vaccine prevents other types of cancer. Research has shown that Gardasil can prevent the development of anal warts which are caused by HPV types 6 and 11. At the moment we don't know whether the vaccine will prevent HPV infection in the mouth. There is research going on to look at the link between HPV and these other types of cancer and how to prevent it.

The HPV vaccination programme

In the UK, girls in Year 8 at school (aged 12 to 13) are offered the HPV vaccine. Girls have three injections over six months. A letter about the vaccine and a consent form is sent to the parents of the girl before she has the vaccine. It is up to her whether she has the vaccine.

From September 2012, the vaccination programme will use Gardasil. This vaccine protects against genital warts as well as cervical cancer.

It is possible to have the vaccination privately. The cost for private treatment varies from doctor to doctor. We are hearing reports of about £400 being charged for a course of three injections.

If girls take up the vaccination at school, the programme will prevent at least seven out of ten cancers of the cervix (70%) and possibly even more in the future. But it takes between ten and 20 years for a cancer to develop after HPV infection. So any benefits in reducing cervical cancer won't be seen for quite a long time. But the number of cases of pre-cancerous changes in the cervix (CIN) will fall quite rapidly.

It is not certain how long the vaccination gives protection for. So far the trials have followed people up for about eight years so we know that it lasts at least this long. It is expected that the vaccines should last for life but more research is needed to find out if this is the case. It may be that women will need a booster dose at some time.

Men and boys and the vaccine

The HPV vaccine is not licensed for men in the UK at the moment. HPV does increase the risk of other types of cancer including penile and anal cancers in men. However, it is not the only cause of these cancers and we don't know how many of these cancers would be prevented by having the vaccine. They are rare cancers and vaccinating all men would be very expensive. It is thought that by vaccinating girls it will reduce the number of men getting HPV because you become infected through sexual contact.

Research into views about HPV

A large project called the HPV (Human Papilloma Virus) Core Messages Study is looking at the scientific evidence about HPV as well as finding out people's views about HPV testing. Based on this, the project aims to develop messages that could help people make informed decisions about HPV testing and vaccination.

If girls are sexually active before having the vaccine

The vaccine is being offered to girls from the age of 12 because they are unlikely to be sexually active and to have caught HPV. The research so far has shown that the vaccine works best at preventing HPV infection in younger women. If you are sexually active before you have the vaccine you may already have HPV and the vaccine won't get rid of it. But there are still benefits from having the vaccine. There are many different types of HPV so even if you have HPV it may not be HPV 16 or 18. Types 16 and 18 are the types that are most likely to cause cancer of the cervix and it is these high-risk types that the vaccines protect against.

If girls become sexually active during the course of the vaccine injections it is important to complete the course of injections. It is only after the three injections that we know the vaccine is protective. However, a recent study in Costa Rica suggested that women who had only two doses of Cervarix may have as much protection from HPV 16 and 18 as those who'd had three doses. But more research is needed before we will know if fewer than three doses gives enough protection and for as long.

Side effects of the vaccine

The side effects are usually mild and include:

⇨ Headache

⇨ Aching muscles

⇨ Redness and soreness around the site of the injection

⇨ Fever

⇨ Feeling and being sick

⇨ Stomach pain

⇨ Diarrhoea

⇨ Itching, rash

⇨ Dizziness.

Do we still need cervical cancer screening?

Yes, we will definitely still need the cervical screening programme in the UK. The vaccines don't prevent infection with all types of HPV. Also from the research so far, we don't think the vaccines will help prevent cervical cancer in women already infected with HPV. And it takes about ten to 20 years after HPV infection for a cervical cancer to develop. So it's very important to remember that women will still need cervical cancer screening (smear tests) for many years to come.

17 September 2012

⇨ The above information is reprinted with kind permission from Cancer Research UK. Taken from CancerHelp UK, the patient information website of Cancer Research UK: http://www.cancerresearchuk.org/cancerhelp.

What is cervical cancer?

Information from NHS Choices.

Cervical cancer is an uncommon type of cancer that develops in a woman's cervix. The cervix is the entrance to the womb from the vagina.

Cervical cancer often has no symptoms in its early stages. If you have symptoms, the most common is unusual vaginal bleeding, which can occur after sex, in between periods or after the menopause.

Abnormal bleeding doesn't mean that you definitely have cervical cancer, but it's a cause for concern. It's important to see your GP as soon as possible. If your GP suspects you might have cervical cancer, you should be referred to see a specialist within two weeks.

'In the UK there were around 950 deaths due to cervical cancer in 2008.'

Screening for cervical cancer

Over the course of many years, the cells lining the surface of the cervix undergo a series of changes. In rare cases, these changed cells can become cancerous. However, cell changes in the cervix can be detected at a very early stage, and treatments can reduce the risk of cervical cancer developing.

The NHS offers a national screening programme for all women over 24 years old. During screening, a small sample of cells is taken from the cervix and checked under a microscope for abnormalities. This test is commonly referred to as a cervical smear test.

It is recommended that women who are between 25 and 49 years old are screened every three years, and women between 50 and 64 are screened every five years. You should be sent a letter telling you when your screening appointment is due. Contact your GP if you think that you may be overdue for a screening appointment.

Treating cervical cancer

If cervical cancer is diagnosed at an early stage, it's usually possible to treat it using surgery. In some cases, it's possible to leave the womb in place, but sometimes it will need to be removed. The surgical procedure that is used to remove the womb is known as a hysterectomy. Radiotherapy is an alternative to surgery for some women with early stage cervical cancer.

More advanced cases of cervical cancer are usually treated using a combination of chemotherapy and radiotherapy. Radiotherapy can also cause infertility as a side effect.

Causes of cervical cancer

Almost all cases of cervical cancer are caused by the human papilloma virus (HPV). HPV is a very common virus that's spread during sex. It's a common cause of genital warts.

There are more than 100 different types of HPV, many of which are harmless. However, some types of HPV can disrupt the normal functioning of the cells of the cervix. This causes them to reproduce uncontrollably and trigger the onset of cancer.

Two distinct strains of the HPV virus are known to be responsible for 70% of all cases of cervical cancer. They are HPV 16 and HPV 18. Most women who are infected with these two types of HPV are unaffected, which means that there must be additional factors that make some women more vulnerable to HPV infection than others.

HPV vaccination

In 2008, a national vaccination programme was launched to vaccinate girls against HPV 16 and HPV 18. The vaccine is most effective if it's given a few years before a girl becomes sexually active, so it's given to girls between the ages of 12 and 13.

The vaccine used is Gardasil – which provides protection against cervical cancer and genital warts

The vaccine protects against the two strains of HPV responsible for more than 70% of cervical cancers in the UK. However you should still attend your future screening appointments even if you have been vaccinated.

'The vaccine protects against the two strains of HPV responsible for more than 70% of cervical cancers in the UK.'

Complications of cervical cancer

Many women with cervical cancer will have complications. Complications can arise as a direct result of the cancer or as a side effect of treatments such as radiotherapy, surgery and chemotherapy.

Complications that are associated with cervical cancer can range from the relatively minor, such as minor bleeding from the vagina or having to urinate frequently, to being life-threatening, such as severe bleeding from the vagina or kidney failure.

Who is affected by cervical cancer?

Due to the success of the NHS screening programme, cervical cancer is now an uncommon type of cancer in the UK. However, it's still a common cause of cancer-related death in countries that don't offer screening.

It's possible for women of all ages to develop cervical cancer. However, the condition mainly affects sexually active women between 25 and 45 years old. Many women who are affected did not attend their screening appointments.

In 2007, nearly 2,800 cases of cervical cancer were diagnosed in the UK. In addition, about 25,000 cases were diagnosed with a pre-cancerous condition of the cervix called cervical intraepithelial neoplasia (CIN).

Outlook

The stage at which cervical cancer is diagnosed is an important factor in determining a woman's outlook. For example, if the cancer is still at an early stage, the outlook will usually be very good and a complete cure is often possible.

More than 90% of women with stage one cervical cancer will live at least five years after receiving a diagnosis. Many women will live much longer. Researchers used five years as a cut-off point because cancer is unlikely to recur after five years and most women can consider themselves cured after five years.

Around one in three people with the more advanced type of cervical cancer will live at least five years.

Another important factor is a woman's age when cervical cancer first develops. Older women usually have a worse outlook than younger women.

In the UK there were around 950 deaths due to cervical cancer in 2008.

4 October 2011

⇨ The above information is reprinted with kind permission from NHS Choices. Please visit www.nhs.uk for further information.

Cervical cancer jab 'gives youngsters green light for promiscuity', charity LIFE says

An anti-abortion charity that advises the Government on sexual health has stirred controversy after pulling a statement on its website that said the cervical cancer jab 'gives young people another green light to be promiscuous'.

LIFE removed the controversial posting on its website after news that many school girls were being denied the jab, which protects against two strains of the human papilloma virus (HPV) that cause 70% of cases of cervical cancer, and is usually offered to girls aged 12-13.

It said: '[young people] do have choices about how they live their lives and the HPV vaccine suggests they won't be able to control themselves. We should have higher expectations for them and show them more respect, not vaccinate them en masse against STIs.'

However, the charity, which had used the message to back faith schools denying students the jab, said it still stood by its statement despite removing it.

Mark Bhagwandin told *The Huffington Post*: 'We still hold fast the comments that we made in that statement, it's just because we are looking at what we do as the media team in terms of what issues we speak on.'

Last week *GP* magazine had found 24 schools in 83 of England's 152 primary care trust (PCT) areas were opting out of the vaccination programme, many of them on religious grounds.

Labour's shadow public health minister Diane Abbott is now calling for Andrew Lansley to remove the group from the Department of Health's Sexual Health Forum, saying their views were 'staggering'.

'It's not good enough to just remove this statement from their website and pretend everything is OK again, because this group is closely advising Andrew Lansley on sexual health policy, and driving this Government's public health agenda,' she said.

'LIFE has an array of policy positions that I find staggering, and it is not suitable for this group to be advising the Government like this,' she said.

In a later statement, LIFE said: 'We wish to emphasise that LIFE was not directed to pull the press release on the HPV vaccine from our website. We decided to withdraw the release because we were concerned that it could be misconstrued or read out of context.

'All those involved in relationships and sex education should think very carefully about the messages being sent about sexual behaviour. For instance, we should be very aware of the danger of giving a false sense of security with measures like the HPV vaccine, which protects only against one particular STI and provides no protection against pregnancy.'

A Department of Health spokesperson told *The Huffington Post*: 'LIFE is one of the 11 groups that sit on the Sexual Health Forum. It is important to ensure that a wide range of views and interests are represented.

'The Sexual Health Forum does not advise on immunisation – this is provided by the independent Joint

Committee on Vaccination and Immunisation.'

The row comes in the wake of continuing controversy over the role of anti-abortion groups in advising the Government.

Last week, *The Huffington Post* revealed anti-abortion charity Lovewise was teaching school children around England that terminations can lead to infection, holes in the womb and dramatically increase the risk of depression and suicide.

LIFE, alongside Lovewise, are members of the Sex and Relationships Education (SRE) council, which was launched in Parliament in May 2011. Education Secretary Michael Gove sent a message of support at the body's launch, saying: 'I look forward to working with you all in ensuring that the interests of families are put at the heart of our policies.'

In a blog for *The Huffington Post*, the chief executive of the Family Planning Association Julie Bentley, who also sits on the Sexual Health Forum, wrote: 'To refuse to offer a vaccine that would protect girls from a life-threatening illness is at best spectacularly

thoughtless, at worst wilfully dangerous.

'It does not recognise that HPV can be passed on through non-penetrative sexual acts such as intimate touching and petting.'

Brook's Chief Executive Simon Blake said: 'It is important that the Sexual Health Forum strives to sustain the progress made in reducing teenage conceptions and not go back to a time when the young had really poor sexual and relationships education and see a rise in teenage pregnancy rates and sexually transmitted infections as a result.

'Brook will continue to work within our pro-choice values and respond to the evidence base in our role on the forum'

The other members of the sexual health forum advising the Government are the Family Planning Association; the British Association for Sexual Health and HIV; the Faculty of Sexual and Reproductive Health at the Royal College of Obstetricians and Gynaecologists; the Association of Directors of Public Health; the British HIV Association; the Terrence Higgins Trust; Brook; the Sex Education Forum; National Children's Bureau and Marie Stopes International.

Compare and contrast

LIFE's original statement

The pro-life education charity, LIFE, says that at face-value, the decision by some faith schools to deny their girls the HPV vaccine seems counterintuitive. However, when given proper thought, the vaccine is yet another measure which treats the symptoms of rising STI rates, not the causes.

A LIFE spokeswoman says:

'Of course, any intervention which promises to prevent cancer is instantly attractive. But let's not forget that we are talking about vaccinating children en masse against sexually transmitted infection and, like it or not, this does send the message that sex can be consequence-free.

'The vaccine has to be considered in the wider context of other messages given to young people from a very young age – sex with multiple partners is OK as long as you use a condom; unwanted pregnancy can be dealt with by taking the morning-after pill; saving sex for a long-term relationship is unrealistic these days and abortion is a woman's right. These are very powerful messages indeed.

'While the vaccine alone may not fuel promiscuity, combined with today's value-free sex education and media messages, it gives young people another 'green light' to be promiscuous. And apart from the risk of other STIs and teen pregnancy, there is as yet no vaccine against the emotional damage to young people which accompanies casual sex.

'LIFE is non-religious charity which runs an education programme around the UK, encouraging young people to think for themselves about sex and relationships. We ask them what will make them truly happy for the long-term, and many are relieved to discuss more life-affirming ways of living than is offered to them in today's culture.

'Young people want to be respected and loved, not used and cast aside. They do have choices about

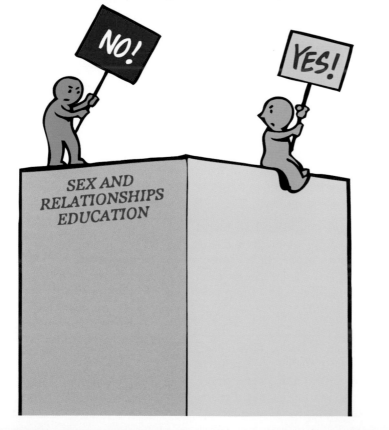

how they live their lives and the HPV vaccine suggests they won't be able to control themselves. We should have higher expectations for them and show them more respect, not vaccinate them en masse against STIs.'

What they say now

LIFE spokesman Mark Bhagwandin said: 'To be absolutely clear: we are not opposed to the HPV vaccine, but we do think that there are legitimate concerns about how well the HPV vaccine integrates with the broader aims and purpose of relationships and sex education, i.e. there is a risk of mixed messages about whether we regard teenage sexual activity as sensible or healthy. Use of this vaccine must be part of a broad, responsible programme of relationships and sex education. It is a wise and sensible measure insofar as many – though far from all – teenagers are going to be sexually active.

'All those involved in relationships and sex education should think very carefully about the messages being sent about sexual behaviour. For instance, we should be very aware of the danger of giving a false sense of security with measures like the HPV vaccine, which protects only against one particular STI and provides no protection against pregnancy.

'Ms Abbott claims that she finds many of our "policy positions" to be "staggering", but fails to be specific about particulars. If she were more constructive, we might be able to open up a fruitful dialogue about achieving the best outcomes for teenage sexual health.'

25 July 2012

⇨ The above information is from *The Huffington Post* and is reprinted with kind permission from AOL (UK). Please visit www.huffingtonpost.co.uk for further information.

Life-saving vaccine denied to girls

Information from Education for Choice.

When the UK Government first decided to provide the human papilloma virus (HPV) vaccine to all girls it was met with opposition from those who claimed that it would 'fuel promiscuity'. Of course this is nonsense and everyone who works in sexual health with young people said so at the time.

Either the vaccinations would be given with no explanation to the girls of the fact that HPV is a sexually transmitted infection in which case most girls would make no connection – either positive or negative – between the vaccine and sexual activity OR – obviously the option we favoured – the vaccination programme would be used as an opportunity to do some sexual health promotion. This work would:

⇨ celebrate the fact that this vaccine could prevent the majority of deaths from cervical cancer

⇨ encourage girls to have regular pap or 'smear' tests once they are old enough

⇨ talk about minimising risk factors for other cancers and the importance of regular breast checks for adult women and testicular checks for men

⇨ outline the risks for men of contracting HPV

⇨ emphasise that the vaccination does not give them protection against any of the other panoply of STIs or, of course, against pregnancy.

I haven't found much information about what education or information is being provided alongside the vaccination, but a recent study published by Elsevier suggests that offering and giving the vaccine has NOT changed young women's sexual behaviour, turned them into wild nymphomaniacs, or caused

them to throw their condoms on the bonfire and caution to the wind.

Today, an article in *The Guardian* reports on schools that are not providing the vaccination because 'their pupils follow strict Christian principles and do not have sex outside marriage'. So, first the vaccination was rejected because it would promote unsafe sexual behaviour and now it is rejected because pupils in some schools don't need it as they will definitely not have sex outside of marriage.

Even if it was true that girls who

> **'Celebrate the fact that this vaccine could prevent the majority of deaths from cervical cancer.'**

commit to chastity in their early teens don't ever end up having pre-marital or extra-marital sex (clue: it isn't), it doesn't take account of the fact that an abstinent girl can be raped, can be coerced into sex, or can marry a man who has previously had sex and is infected with HPV.

Approximately 1,000 women in the UK die each year from cervical cancer. Clearly the schools that are rejecting the vaccination think that this is a risk worth taking...

18 July 2012

⇨ Information from Education for Choice. Please visit www.educationforchoice.blogspot.co.uk and www.efc.org.uk for further information.

New study reveals extent of Jade Goody effect on cervical screening

Information from NHS Cancer Screening Programmes.

Three years ago, Jade Goody died of cervical cancer. A new study, published today in the _Journal of Medical Screening_, discusses the effect of her death on cervical screening attendance. It showed that more than 400,000 extra women were screened in England between mid-2008 and mid-2009 – the period during which Jade Goody was diagnosed and died of cervical cancer.

More women of all ages were screened, though the increase was greater for women aged under 50. In the 25-29 age group, an estimated 31,000 extra women were screened in the five months between autumn 2008 and spring 2009. It seems that the women who were closest to Jade Goody in age or circumstances,

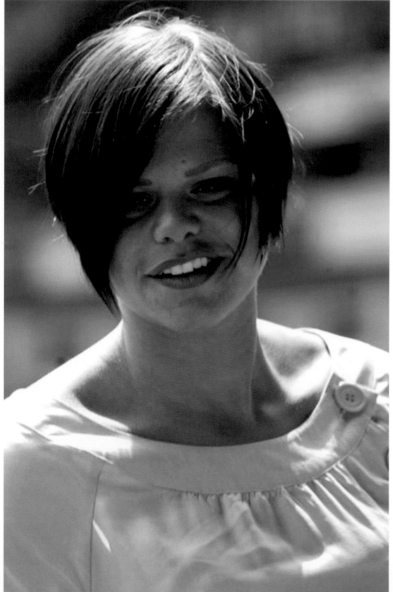

that is young women with young families, were those most affected by her experience.

Although there was concern that the increase in attendance might have been from the 'worried well' coming back for an early repeat screen, the research found that the opposite was true. A higher proportion was from women who were late for their test, rather than those who were coming back early. In the 25-49 age group, for example, 82,000 (28 per cent) women had not been tested for five years or longer, while only 7,500 (eight per cent) were coming back early having already been screened in the past three years.

Professor Julietta Patnick, Director of the NHS Cancer Screening Programmes, commented;

'Jade's tragic diagnosis and death played a huge role in raising awareness of cervical cancer and prompted a welcome increase in screening attendance in 2008/2009. Many of those women will now be due their next routine appointment and we would like to see them return.

'All women between the ages of 25 and 64 are eligible for free cervical screening every three to five years. Regular screening means that changes in the cervix which may develop into cancer can be identified and treated. Screening saves lives, and we would encourage all eligible women to consider attending a screening appointment when invited.

'It is important to remember, however, that cervical screening is aimed at women without symptoms. Women of any age with symptoms (for example, bleeding between periods or after intercourse) should contact their GP or genito-urinary medicine (GUM) clinic who will refer them to see an expert in hospital.'

1 June 2012

⇨   The above information is reprinted with kind permission from NHS Cancer Screening Programmes. Please visit www.cancerscreening.nhs.uk for further information.

Sex education

The UK still has a worryingly high teenage pregnancy rate, and sexually transmitted infections are also on the rise. Is sex education – or the lack of it – in schools to blame? We look at the facts of life...

By Kia Henson

There's something wrong with sex education in this country. There must be. The results speak for themselves. The highest number of teenage pregnancies in the whole of Western Europe (45, 873 in 2008). 20,000 girls under 18 undergoing an abortion last year. And high numbers of sexually transmitted infections (STIs); recent figures show 15- to 24-year-olds are still the group most affected by STIs in the UK. Dr Gwenda Hughes, head of the Health Protection Agency's STI section, says: 'The impact of STI diagnoses is still unacceptably high in this group. Studies suggest those infected may be more likely to have unsafe sex or lack the skills and confidence to negotiate safer sex.' Perhaps the 'relationships' aspect of Sex and Relationships Education (SRE) is seriously lacking.

Results from a campaign called Let's Talk About Sex, set up by 18-year-old Shereece Marcantonio, indicate that 40% of young people believe their sex education was poor. Shereece's campaign, run in conjunction with Channel 4's *Battlefront*, Campaigners on a Mission (www.battlefront.co.uk/sex) aims for a change in the way sex education is taught in schools: this young woman, whose three siblings all became teenage parents, wants to establish peer-to-peer sex education in schools, whereby young people are trained up to become educators so they

can teach each other about sex. Her mission? To ensure young people can 'get the facts they need without the cringe'. She wants this vital subject taught 'in a language that teenagers all understand' – and to reverse the UK's shocking teen pregnancy, STI and abortion rates. Shereece is now a qualified sex and relationships educator who delivers lessons to secondary school children in east London and Essex. Shereece adds: 'It's all got to be about safe sex.'

Where does the problem lie?

A brief (and very unofficial) vox pop on SRE highlighted several issues. 'Traumatised.' One mum's analysis of her son's reaction to his first SRE lesson in Year Five. 'Terrified.' Another mum's description of her ten-year-old daughter's reaction to a video of a live birth. 'Outdated and corny.' A teacher's verdict of the video used in her lesson. 'It scared me and made me not want to use any. We were just told all about the bad side effects.' One teenage girl's opinion after a Year Nine lesson about contraception. 'Strange and vague.' A teenage girl's response to seeing a cartoon on the subject at primary school. And secondary school, where it's part of PSHE (Personal, Social, Health and Economic Education) was no better for her: 'Totally forgettable PowerPoint slides.'

It's little wonder, then, that guest editor Dr Christian considers sex

education 'shoddy', and blames it for our poor sexual health.

SRE is, shockingly, not compulsory in schools. All schools are required to have a policy on it, but that policy could, in fact, be not to teach it. Brook (www.brook.org.uk), a charity that provides free, confidential advice to people under 25, says children face a 'lottery' over how much SRE they are taught. Statistics from Brook show that one in four children get no SRE at all. And of those that do, 80% say they 'have no voice in what they learn'. Even in lessons given, young people say they 'don't learn enough about emotions and relationships'. The figures also show that 36% of children claim to learn the most from friends their own age – which means it could be inaccurate – and, most worrying of all, a mere 7% claim to learn from their parents.

Models to learn from

Perhaps UK teachers, and parents, need to learn a few lessons from the Dutch. The Netherlands has the lowest rate of teenage pregnancy in Europe. Sex education in Holland is not required to follow a national curriculum, so teachers are able to teach about sex in many different ways. Indeed, Shereece's *Battlefront* study revealed that 'pupils empathise better with a more creative approach to sex and relationships education'. Parents back up school education, too – the country's culture of tolerance and pragmatism allows children to talk openly about sexuality with their parents at home. Scenes of British families discussing sex over the dinner table are, sadly, a long way off. Sex is still regarded as taboo when it comes to family conversation.

In addition, the Dutch approach has a heavy focus on empowerment and respect – put simply, the importance of being able to say, 'no'. We're not talking abstinence, but how to deal with pressure. Teaching looks at the seriousness of sex in relation to consent, the significance of first sexual intercourse and, crucially, potential pregnancy.

Findings from the UK Data Archive's *National Survey of Sexual Attitudes and Lifestyles* revealed that, of those surveyed, one in five young men and almost half of young women between the ages of 16 and 24 wished they had waited longer to start having sex. Anyone who had intercourse under the age of 15 was twice as likely to wish they'd waited. With today's figures,

it seems it's a case of after the horse has bolted...

Sweden follows a similar style of sex education to Holland. Lessons start from the age of six – covering anatomy, eggs and sperm; from age 12, the focus moves to disease, contraception, moral issues and gender equality. And it works: teen pregnancies, seven per 1,000 births, and STI rates are both among the world's lowest.

Nurse-led lessons

Do children feel more engaged when taught by a healthcare professional?

An interesting fact was revealed in the *Battlefront* research – 48% of girls said they'd like to be taught by a doctor or nurse (compared to 38% of boys).

From our own vox pop, Amy, 16, said: 'When our school nurse came to talk to us, it was more useful and interesting than when the teacher taught us. She knew much more

on the topic and interacted with the class – she mainly talked about sexual health and contraception. It was easier having someone who was more like a visitor, and she chatted with us on a more personal level. Without her, I wouldn't have learnt so much and I felt more comfortable asking her questions.'

But comments from Grace, 14, who also had nurse-led lessons, still favour 'age' over 'medical knowledge': 'In Year Nine we had a lesson about contraception and pregnancy. That wasn't very good at all. We had a nurse in but it would have been much better if it was a younger woman who we could relate to; I would have felt more comfortable and would have asked about more things I was unsure about.'

Shereece adds: 'Peer educators are not trying to replace teachers, but combined together, perhaps with sexual health services and doctor or nurse-led classes, there would be a fantastic compilation of quality SRE.' One simple fact can't be contested. We learn more when we like the way we're being taught. For that reason alone, a change in sex education can't come soon enough. Perhaps creativity is core: bin the slide shows and start thinking carrots and condoms. That might be food for thought.

If you want to show your support for Shereece's campaign, go to www.battlefront.co.uk/sex to add your name to her campaign. As we went to print, there were currently 4,580 supporters. Or visit www.brook.co.uk and sign its petition for the Government, demanding 21st Century Sex and Relationships Education.

4 April 2012

⇨ The above information is reprinted with kind permission from EMP PLC. Originally published in *At Home* magazine (www.athomemagazine.co.uk).

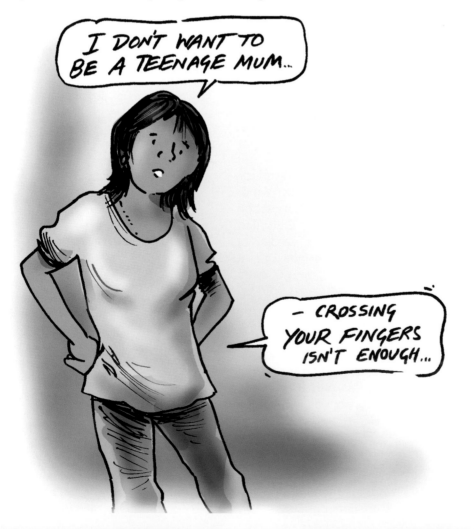

UK sex and relationships education fails to prepare young people for modern day life

Information from Brook.

Almost half (47%) of today's secondary school pupils say Sex and Relationships Education (SRE) doesn't cover what they really need to know about sex.

The information void this creates isn't filled by parents – only 5% of young people get their information from their mum and 1% from their dad.

82% of young people say schools should listen to young people when shaping SRE.

New research released today shows 47% of secondary school pupils think their school's Sex and Relationships Education (SRE) does not meet their needs. The lack of relevant sex and relationships education in schools and at home means 81% of teenagers are getting most of their sexual health knowledge from less reliable sources, leaving them vulnerable and ill-prepared to navigate their way through relationships.

The study of over 2,000 14-18-year-olds, commissioned by Brook, the country's largest young people's sexual health charity illustrates the impact on young people that the country's lack of commitment to good Sex and Relationships Education, out of date guidelines for schools and a lack of support for well qualified teachers is having.

The survey finds that young people rely on often ill-informed sources, such as peers, for information resulting in the spread of dangerous sex myths which can lead to poor decisions and unwanted outcomes. The five most commonly shared sex myths amongst peers are:

⇨ 59% of young people have wrongly heard from their friends that a woman cannot get pregnant if the man withdraws before he ejaculates.

⇨ 58% of young people have wrongly heard that women cannot get pregnant if they are having their period.

⇨ 35% have wrongly heard that women cannot get pregnant if they have sex standing up.

⇨ 33% have wrongly heard from their friends that a woman cannot get pregnant if it is the first time she has had sex.

⇨ 25% of young people have wrongly heard that you can only catch HIV from gay sex.

Schools are not required to consult with their pupils to shape SRE lessons, and 78% of young people confirm they have never been consulted. As the Government recently announced a review of Personal, Social, Health and Economic Education (PSHE), 82% of young people said they want schools to take their views into account to help make SRE relevant for the 21st century.

The research identified the scale of the SRE problem:

⇨ One in four (26%) secondary pupils get no SRE in school whatsoever.

⇨ A quarter (26%) of those who do get SRE say the teacher isn't able to teach it well.

⇨ Only 13% of 14-18-year-olds learn most about sex from their SRE teacher, and just 5% from Mum and 1% from dad at home.

⇨ The sex information void is being filled by friends their own age (36%), their boyfriend/girlfriend (10%), TV programmes (8%) and online porn (5%) – none of which are reliable sources of honest, useful information.

⇨ SRE fares particularly badly when it comes to teaching pupils about relationships, with only 6% saying they get the information on relationships that they need in SRE lessons.

In light of this research, Brook is launching the 'Say YES to 21st Century Sex and Relationships Education' campaign to give today's teenagers their say on how they want to be taught SRE and what they want to learn, as part of its wider Sex:Positive work. Over the next seven weeks, Brook will gather the views of thousands more young people and present its resulting report to the Department for Education, ahead of the submissions deadline for its review into SRE as part of PSHE.

Jules Hillier, Brook Deputy Chief Executive, says:

'Young people in Britain deserve honest, useful information about sex and relationships but SRE in UK schools is failing them. Standards vary so widely that all too often young people miss out on the information they need to stay safe, healthy and happy. Worse, we know that the void is not being filled by reliable information from elsewhere – like parents – but from the playground and, even more worrying, Internet porn.

'Learning about sex and relationships is a crucial life skill and by letting teenagers leave school ill-informed we are letting them down. We are calling on young people to seize the opportunity to make their voices heard by telling us what they think 21st century SRE should cover, to better meet their needs.'

Yessica, Brook volunteer said:

'My school didn't offer SRE classes until Year 11, when I was 15 going on 16, by which time I was pregnant so it was too late. I wasn't allowed to take part in the lessons as the teacher said it wouldn't be relevant for me, so I had to look elsewhere for information which was often incorrect.

'I do not blame my school for my decisions but if I was taught SRE sooner and had been given honest, accurate information when I needed it, I would have had a different mentality and would have made different choices. That is why Brook's "Say YES to 21st Century Sex and Relationships Education" campaign is so important to me.'

To support Brook's 'Say YES to 21st Century Sex and Relationships Education' campaign sign up to the petition here: http://www.change. org/petitions/uk-parliament-support-21st-century-sex-and-relationship-education.

For more information about the campaign, please visit http://www.brook.org.uk/sex-positive.

Show support of the 'Say YES to 21st Century Sex and Relationships Education' campaign via Twitter, using the hashtags #sexednevertaughtme and #whatsexedtaughtme.

Research

All figures quoted in the release are from ResearchBods (formerly Dubit) 'Direct to Youth' research panel. Total sample size was 2,029 14-18-year-olds and the figures are representative of all young people in the UK. All panel members under the age of 16 have the express verbal and recorded consent of their parent or guardian to participate. Fieldwork was undertaken between 14-28 September 2011.

12 October 2011

⇨ The above information is reprinted with kind permission from Brook. Please visit www.brook.org.uk for further information.

© *Brook*

Explicit sex education website condemned as 'grossly irresponsible'

NHS and council officials have been accused of 'condoning' sexual experimentation among under-age teenagers after creating a website and mobile phone app featuring explicit sex tips for children as young as 13.

By Sam Marsden

The free online service features pictures of a naked man and woman with their erogenous zones highlighted, a 'sextionary' including definitions of slang terms for genitalia, and a question-and-answer section covering a variety of sexual acts.

A family charity said the Respect Yourself website, which is modelled on the more liberal Dutch approach to sex education, was 'grossly irresponsible' and encouraged an 'unhealthy obsession with physical acts'.

The Internet site and smartphone app, the first of their kind in Britain, are aimed at children 13 and over, and were created by a team from Warwickshire County Council working with NHS Warwickshire and Coventry University.

An FAQ section features answers to questions posed by teenagers ranging from 'What is the most common age to lose your virginity?' to 'Where can I buy the *Kama Sutra*?'.

In response to the question, 'Why do you have to be 16 to have sex? What if you want it now?', the website states: 'The law says you are not old enough to decide for yourself until you are 16 – as this is the age the law sees us as being mature enough to decide. You are the only one who knows when you are ready. Some are ready before, some not till much later.'

Young people thinking about losing their virginity are directed to a page entitled 'Am I Ready?' with a list of six questions designed to help them decide.

The £24,000 cost of developing the site and app came from an NHS West Midlands research fund.

Norman Wells, director of the Family Education Trust, a national charity, claimed that the website only 'paid lip service' to the legal age of consent, adding: 'It pretty much tells young people they can engage in sexual activity whenever they feel ready, regardless of what the law says.'

He went on: 'Parents throughout the region will be appalled that health professionals have supported the development of a resource that condones sexual experimentation by young people and uses crude and sometimes even foul language.

'This is a grossly irresponsible website and a complete misuse of taxpayers' hard-earned cash.

'Many of the topics covered are totally unnecessary and positively unhelpful. Young people – and older people for that matter – simply don't need a 'sextionary' containing an A-Z of all manner of sexual practices and perversions.

'It merely encourages an unhealthy obsession with physical acts and will do nothing to help young people build healthy relationships or prepare them for a stable and fulfilling marriage in the future.

'Not only does the site include a considerable volume of unhealthy and unhelpful content, but much of the information provided is not even accurate.'

The website's developers used research from a European-funded study tour of the Netherlands, where sex education for young people focuses on pleasure as well as biological facts.

Amy Danahay, project manager of Respect Yourself, said: 'The Internet has changed how young people find out about sex.

'It would be naïve to think that many young people are not regularly accessing far more explicit material and if we want to give them access to relevant information, we have to move with the times – 53 per cent of ten-year-olds have accessed some kind of porn on the Internet.

'It is far better that we provide accurate information for them which is easily accessible and monitored by professionals.

'We have involved young people throughout the development about how best to reach them and communicate with them. We have used language that young people understand and use. The app has been based on thorough research into what young people need, how they want to access the information and how it should be presented.

'It is based on research into how this information is presented in Holland where the rate of teenage pregnancy is over five times lower than it is in England and where contraception is much more widely used. Clearly their approach has worked and we would be wrong if we neglected to take lessons from that.'

24 October 2012

⇨ The above article originally appeared in *The Telegraph* and is reprinted with permission. Please visit www.telegraph.co.uk for further information.

Sex education: we should teach young people about more than the mechanics

Young people need comprehensive sexuality education, which will help them make more informed decisions.

By Doortje Braeken

Sex education polarises opinion, sets legislators against parents and parents against schools and regularly inflames media opinion. Somewhere in the middle sit young people: ill-served, receiving confused messages and gaining their information from famously unreliable sources, such as peers or the Internet.

Sex education, as all too many experience it, is like teaching people how to drive by telling them in detail what's under the bonnet, how the bits work, how to maintain them safely to avoid accidents, what the controls do and when to go on the road. It's all about the mechanics. And that's it.

There's a growing consensus that young people don't need sex education, they need comprehensive sexuality education (CSE). CSE is sex education plus: the mechanics, plus a lots more about sexuality.

That means not just teaching young people about the biology of sex, but also teaching them about the personal, emotional, societal and cultural forces which shape the way in which they choose to conduct their lives. Armed with this understanding, young people can make far more considered decisions.

This approach has the potential to unite the warring factions that bicker over the fundamental rights and wrongs of sex education: CSE equips young people with basic biological knowledge, but at the same time it equips them to question why they act in certain ways, and whether or not it is right, valuable or desirable to do so. CSE imparts information, and promotes responsibility.

CSE contains components which allow learners to explore and discuss gender, and the diverse spectrum of gender identities that exist within and between and beyond simple heterosexuality. It also contains components that examine the dynamics of power in relationships, and individual rights.

These are not taught as theoretical concepts. They have serious practical effects on the way in which young people interact with each other, both in the sexual and the wider social and educational spheres. Studies have shown that addressing such issues can have a marked impact both in school and the expansion of young people's social networks.

CSE also engages with what some doubtless regard as difficult territory. Sexuality – however, individually, we choose to regard it – is a critical aspect of personal identity. The pleasure that we derive from sexuality, even if that pleasure is the pleasure of feeling that a reproductive duty is being fulfilled, is a vital part of our lives: it's what makes us human. CSE views sexuality as a positive force.

CSE exploits a variety of teaching and learning techniques that are respectful of age, experience and cultural backgrounds, and which engage young people by enabling them to personalise the information they receive.

What is most telling is that a large number

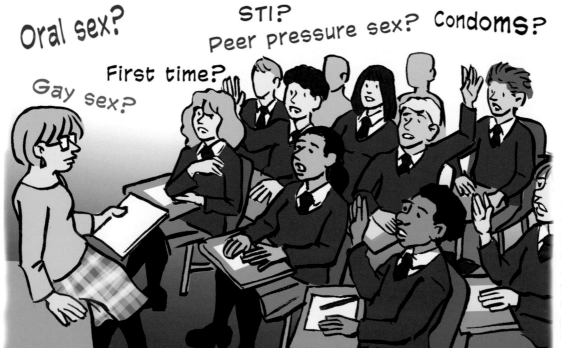

Oral sex? STI? Peer pressure sex? Condoms? First time? Gay sex?

of studies have reached the clear conclusion that CSE does not lead to earlier sexual initiation or an increase in sexual activity. To paraphrase, traditional sex education seems to say: 'If you're going to do it, this is how everything works and you need to protect yourself in these ways to prevent this.' CSE says all that, but it also asks young people to ponder what exactly 'it' is, and to deepen their perception of its implications.

In a political environment which is quantitatively driven, we measure the success of sex education in straightforward health behaviour indicators. These are easy to manage: numbers which build on existing health surveillance and measurement systems, and which are simple to understand from an objective point of view.

However, CSE is a far more nuanced discipline, and it will be necessary to include other measures of programme success: qualitative, subjective indicators which relate to gender equity, empowerment and critical thinking skills.

While governments have recognised young people's right to CSE via various intergovernmental resolutions and conventions, the journey from recognition to delivery will be a long one. Even in the UK, there are notable differences, with England having a bare-bones biological approach 'puberty, menstruation, contraception, abortion, safer sex, HIV/Aids and STIs should be covered', while Wales and Scotland have curriculums which incline far more towards the CSE agenda.

The International Planned Parenthood Federation, the organisation I work for, and its 153 member associations around the world, has been instrumental in pressing for the adoption of international policy commitments to CSE. For many, it may seem like we are pushing ten steps ahead of the agenda when the basic principle of young people's right to even the most basic introduction to the biology of sex is still not universally accepted.

Our view is different: it is that CSE is what will secure widespread acceptance of sex education, because it is about more than the mechanics of sex. It is about helping young people the world over to become more healthy, more informed, more respectful and more active participants in the life of their community and their nation.

24 May 2012

⇨ The above information originally appeared in *The Guardian* and is reprinted with permission. Please visit www.guardian.co.uk for further information.

Teenagers want sex education from their peers, study finds

Young people are turning to friends for sex and relationships (SRE) education because teachers 'come up short', latest research has found.

By Neil Puffett

A ComRes survey of schools around Britain for Channel 4 shows half of 13- to 17-year-olds questioned (49 per cent) felt they had received too little SRE in their schools.

The majority of pupils (56 per cent) said they are most likely to learn about sex from their friends. And 82 per cent of the 1,123 questioned wanted sex and relationships education to come from a trained young person.

The survey suggests current SRE lessons are not meeting young people's needs. The Government is due to publish an Internal review of personal, social, health and economic education on 30 November.

The poll found that half (49 per cent) of pupils felt awkward asking questions in SRE lessons taught by teachers – only one in five felt comfortable asking questions.

But 67 per cent of pupils said they would be comfortable asking questions to a trained young person.

In total 70 per cent wanted to receive more SRE lessons taught by a trained young person compared to three per cent who didn't.

Shereece Marcantonio, an 18-year-old peer sex and relationships educator from east London, has been campaigning for teenagers to be taught by trained older teenagers.

She said: 'My campaign has always been about changing the national curriculum, by trying to get peer-to-peer teaching of sex and relationship education.

'If we can educate kids in a relaxed and engaging way, we can help avoid unwanted pregnancies and help teenagers cope with their first sexual experiences safely.'

16 November 2011

⇨ The above information is reprinted with kind permission from Children and Young People Now. Please visit www.cypnow.co.uk for further information.

Key facts

⇨ There is also a form of contraception called the emergency contraception pill, which can help prevent unintended pregnancy. It can be taken by girls within 72 hours after unprotected sex, although preferably with 24 hours. It is available across the counter at chemists or from your local GP, family planning clinic or sexual health clinic. (page 2)

⇨ There's a myth that a girl can't get pregnant if she has sex during her period. The truth is, she can get pregnant at any time of the month if she has sex without contraception. (page 3)

⇨ The male condom is 98% effective if it is used according to instructions. This means that two women in 100 will get pregnant in a year. (page 6)

⇨ If 100 sexually active women don't use any contraception, 80 to 90 will become pregnant in a year. (page 6)

⇨ In Brazil and Indonesia, where there is limited sex education, as many as 67% and 48% of young people have a close friend of family member who has had an unplanned pregnancy. Furthermore, in France and Norway, where 85% and 84% of young people receive sex education, only 25% and 24%, know a close friend or family member who has had an unplanned pregnancy. (page 8)

⇨ 44% of young people prioritise personal hygiene, including showering, waxing and applying perfume, above contraception when preparing for a date that may lead to sex. (page 9)

⇨ If unmet need for contraception was fully satisfied, each year 53 million more unintended pregnancies could be prevented. (page 10)

⇨ 15% of young adults between the ages of 18 and 26 have had a sexually transmitted disease in the past year. (page 10)

⇨ Having sex without gaining consent could potentially lead to you spending up to eight years in prison. (page 13)

⇨ The results of the 2011 Young Life and Times survey show that nearly three quarters of 16-year-olds had not had sex. Among those who did, almost half said having sex for them was a natural follow-on in the relationship they were in at the time. (page 17)

⇨ The best way to avoid STIs is to use a condom every time you have sex. (page 18)

⇨ The most common STI in the UK is chlamydia. About seven in ten infected women and half of infected men won't have any obvious signs or symptoms of chlamydia. (page 20)

⇨ A new survey from The Site.org revealed that 16- to 25-year-olds have a worrying lack of concern about the dangers of STIs, with almost half (47%) of respondents agreeing that it's OK to have sex without a condom, providing the girl is on the pill. (page 23)

⇨ In 2008, a national vaccination programme was launched to vaccinate girls against HPV 16 and HPV 18. The vaccine is most effective if it's given a few years before a girl becomes sexually active, so it's given to girls between the ages of 12 and 13. The vaccine used is Gardasil – which provides protection against cervical cancer and genital warts. The vaccine protects against the two strains of HPV responsible for more than 70% of cervical cancers in the UK. (page 28)

⇨ Approximately 1,000 women in the UK die each year from cervical cancer. (page 31)

⇨ Almost half (47%) of today's secondary school pupils say Sex and Relationships Education (SRE) doesn't cover what they really need to know about sex. (page 35)

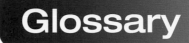

Cervical cancer

Cancer that develops in a woman's cervix (the entrance to the womb from the vagina). In its early stages it often has no symptoms. Symptoms can include unusual vaginal bleeding which can occur after sex, in between periods or after menopause. The NHS offers a national screening programme; a 'smear test' for all women over 24 years old.

Condoms

A thin rubber (latex) sleeve worn on the penis. When used correctly, condoms are the only form of contraception that protect against pregnancy AND STIs. They are 98% effective – this means that two out of 100 women using male condoms as contraception will become pregnant in one year. You can get free condoms from sexual health clinics and some GP surgeries.

Contraception

Sometimes called birth control, contraception is a way to prevent pregnancy. Some forms of contraception, but not all, help reduce the spread of STIs. Contraception is a very important part of making sure sex is safe and taking responsibility for your actions. There are many different types of contraception available; such as the pill, condoms, diaphragms, contraceptive implant (e.g. Implanon) and contraceptive injections.

Contraceptive implant

A small flexible tube about the size of a matchstick inserted by a doctor under the skin of a female's upper arm. The device releases hormones to prevent the ovaries from releasing eggs. Lasts for three years, but can be removed before then if the woman decided she wants to get pregnant.

Contraceptive injections

An injection offers eight to 12 weeks protection against pregnancy, but not from sexually transmitted diseases (approx. 99% effective). It works by thickening the mucus in the cervix, which stops sperm reaching the egg, and it also thins the lining of the womb so that an egg can't implant itself there.

Diaphragms

A rubber dome-shaped device worn inside the vagina which creates a seal against the walls of the vagina. It must be inserted before sexual intercourse and must remain in places for up to six to eight hours afterwards. The diaphragm does not provide protection from sexually transmitted diseases.

Emergency contraception

Sometimes referred to as the 'morning-after pill', this is a form of emergency contraception which can be taken by girls within 72 hours after unprotected sex (although preferably within the first 24 hours). It should not be used as a regular method of contraceptive. It is available across the counter at chemists or from your local GP, family planning clinic or sexual health clinic.

Femidom

Female condom: used by the female partner to provide a physical barrier that prevents sperm from reaching the egg. Can help prevent pregnancy and reduce the risk of STIs.

HPV vaccination

An injection for girls which can help prevent cervical cancer and genital warts. The vaccine protects against the two strains of HPV (human papilloma virus) responsible for more than 70% of cervical cancers in the UK. It is most effective a few years before a girl becomes sexually active. A national vaccination programme launched in 2008 to vaccinate 12- and 13-year-old girls.

Safe sex

Being safe with sex means caring for both your own health, and the health of your partner. Being safe protects you from getting or passing on STIs and from unplanned pregnancy.

Sexual health

Taking care of your sexual health means more than being free from sexually transmissible infections (STIs) or not having to face an unplanned pregnancy. It also means taking responsibility for your body, your health, your partner's health and your decisions about sex.

Sexually transmitted infections (STIs / STDs)

A sexually transmitted infection (STIs), also referred to as sexually transferred diseases (STDs), is a bacterial or viral infection that is spread through sexual contact. This doesn't just mean vaginal/anal sexual intercourse, but also oral sex (licking/sucking on someone's genitals) and sexual touching (skin-to-skin contact). Using condoms are the best way of avoiding STIs. Although STIs are treatable, if left unchecked and untreated they may cause serious damage to long-term health, such as infertility. The most common STI in the UK is chlamydia.

The pill

A tablet taken each day, at the same time, by girls to prevent pregnancy. The pill contains hormones that prevent the ovaries from releasing an egg. It only protects against pregnancy and not STIs.

Assignments

1. Create an informative leaflet about the different kinds of sexually transmitted infections (STIs), including how they are passed on, symptoms and how to treat them.

2. In groups, design a storyboard for a series of YouTube videos that will promote the use of contraception amongst young people.

3. Chlamydia is the most common sexually transmitted infection amongst young people. Create an informative presentation on the signs and symptoms of chlamydia, the risks associated with it and how somebody can request a free test kit.

4. 'I won't get pregnant if we have sex standing up' is a common myth that many of us may have heard. What other sexual health related myths have you heard that need busting? Discuss in pairs or small groups, then read '15 things you should know about sex' on page 3 and 'Contraception myths' on page 11. Compare your answers (note: these articles are not a list of ALL the myths and facts regarding sex, only a small selection).

5. Draw a cartoon strip about how to put on and use a condom correctly that would be suitable to be used in sex education lessons for your age-group.

6. Imagine you are a journalist for your local newspaper, read 'New survey reveals young people are unaware of STI risks' on page 23 and write a summary of the article's findings.

7. Your friend has been dating his girlfriend for several months and he has confided in you that he thinks that they are both ready to have sex. Although he is over 16, she is not. He explains that it will be okay because she has given him sexual consent. How do you respond? What do you think he should do?

8. What is the definition of rape? Look at sex and the law in the UK. What are the possible consequences of sex or physical closeness without consent? Consider not just the legal impact, but the health and emotional effects too. Write a summary of your findings.

9. Your friend Jenny has confided in you that, although her partner does not physically force her, she feels pressured into performing sexual acts that she isn't sure about. Although in the past she has consented to having sex, even when she says no they sometimes have sex anyway. How do you respond to Jenny? What advice would you give her?

10. In 2008, a national vaccination programme was launched to vaccinate girls against HPV 16 and HPV 18. Conduct some research and gather information on the HPV vaccination programme and the vaccine itself. Here are a few questions to get you started: What does the vaccine do? Are there any negative side effects or problems? Can males be given the HPV injection?

11. 'Almost half (47%) of today's secondary school pupils say Sex and Relationships Education (SRE) doesn't cover what they really need to know about sex.' ('UK sex and relationships education fails to prepare young people for modern day life' on page 35). Do you agree? How do you feel about the sex education you received at school? How could it be improved upon?

12. Plan a sex education class to be taught to ten- to 12-year olds. What information would you include? What information would you leave out? Who would be best to teach the class (e.g. a younger woman, an experienced nurse, a teacher, a parent)?

13. At what age should sex education be taught? How young is too young? Debate this as a group.

14. Read 'New study reveals extent of Jade Goody effect on cervical screening.' on page 32. What is the 'Jade Goody effect'? What effect did it have on cervical screening? Using this information, create your own cervical cancer awareness campaign. Use the Internet to see if there are any campaigns currently running and look at sexual health awareness campaigns for inspiration too.

15. Sexual health is not just all about STIs; it should also include a respectful understanding of sex and the mental and emotional aspects involved. Make a list of all the things a person should consider before having sexual intercourse.

16. Design a leaflet that will be given to parents of teenage children, offering hints and tips on how they should approach talking about sex and sexual health with their teenager.

Acknowledgements

The publisher is grateful for permission to reproduce the following material.

While every care has been taken to trace and acknowledge copyright, the publisher tenders its apology for any accidental infringement or where copyright has proved untraceable. The publisher would be pleased to come to a suitable arrangement in any such case with the rightful owner.

Chapter One: What is sexual health?

What is sexual health? © The State of Queensland (Queensland Health) 2010, *15 things you should know about sex* © NHS Choices 2011, *Sexual health quiz* © Bedfordshire PCT, *Questions and answers about contraception* © 2012 University of Oxford, *'Clueless or clued up: your right to be informed about contraception' media report* © Bayer HealthCare Pharmaceuticals, *Contraception myths* © 2012 Whittall Street Clinic, *Sexual consent and the law* © Crown copyright 2012, *Messed up?* © 2012 ARK.

Chapter Two: STIs, HPV and cancer

All about STIs © Brook, *Types of STIs* © Bupa 2011, *Chlamydia* © test.me 2010, *New survey reveals young people are unaware of STI risks* © 2012 YouthNet, *Sexually transmitted infection rates soar among young* © Guardian News & Media Ltd 2012, *Condoms: too embarrassed to buy them?* © 2000-2012 YouGov plc, *HPV vaccines* © Cancer Research UK, *What is cervical cancer?* © NHS Choices 2011, *Cervical cancer jab 'gives youngsters green light for promiscuity', charity LIFE says* © 2012 AOL (UK) Limited, *Life-saving vaccine denied to girls* © Education for Choice 2012, *New study reveals extent of Jade Goody effect on cervical screening* © 2000 – 2012 NHS Cancer Screening Programmes.

Chapter Three: Sex education

Sex education © 2009-2012 EMP PLC, *UK sex and relationships education fails to prepare young people for modern day life* © Brook, *Explicit sex education website condemned as 'grossly irresponsible'* © Telegraph Media Group Limited 2012, *Sex education: we should*

teach young people about more than the mechanics © Guardian News & Media Ltd 2012, *Teenagers want sex education from their peers, study finds* © MA Business & Leisure Limited 2012.

Illustrations:

Pages 24, 30: Don Hatcher; pages 18, 38: Angelo Madrid; pages 26, 34: Simon Kneebone.

Images:

Cover: © Dan Comaniciu, page 5 © Pixels Away, page 6 © Julien Tromeur, page 11 © Joe Cicack, page 12 © gabuchia, page 21 © Mark Wragg, page 32 © Keira76, page 35 © CactuSoup.

Additional acknowledgements:

Editorial on behalf of Independence Educational Publishers by Cara Acred.

With thanks to the Independence team: Mary Chapman, Sandra Dennis, Christina Hughes, Jackie Staines and Jan Sunderland.

Cara Acred

Cambridge, January 2013